The
Golf Doc

Health,
Humor,
and
Insight
to Improve
Your Game

After reading *The Golf Doc*, I can't overemphasize the importance of fitness in the modern game of golf. As this book shows, proper physical preparation and preventive care are invaluable when it comes to maintaining your game.

Greg Norman

Golfers of all ages can benefit from the health tips that *The Golf Doc* provides.

Chi Chi Rodriguez

Valuable, practical, and full of humor. . . you'll learn how to prevent injuries, treat common aches and pains, and improve your game—all at the same time.

Dick Hill, Former Senior Tour Player and Senior Instructor at the Dave Pelz Short Game School

This book is vital reading for anyone who plays golf. *The Golf Doc* will save lives on and off the course. It provides insight into proper health and fitness and the benefits of golf in people's lives.

Laura A. Drumm, President, PCA (Professional Caddies Association) Worldwide

This exciting book will help every golfer improve his or her game by staying fit and healthy. *The Golf Doc* is one tool that helps save lives!

Tom Wildenhaus, PGA Golf Professional PGA Education Committee, South Florida Section

The Golf Doc is an excellent collection of "curbside consults." The information is accurate and nearly encyclopedic. Who knows, maybe it will decrease the number of times physicians are stopped on the fairway with, 'Hey Doc, you got a minute?' It should be in every avid golfer's bag.

Michael Jon Cohen, MD,
Vascular Surgeon, Avid Golfer, and President/Founder, Inside Right, Inc.

What fun, entertaining, and informative reading! It's great to know we now have good, solid, fun information to share in order to help caddies worldwide stay healthy. *The Golf Doc* truly hits home and will help preserve the tradition of caddies in the game.

Dennis M. Cone, Founder, PCA Worldwide.com

The Golf Doc presents a complete and lively compendium of everything you wanted to know about your health on the golf course.

Marlyn Varcoe, Ph.D., Sports Psychologist

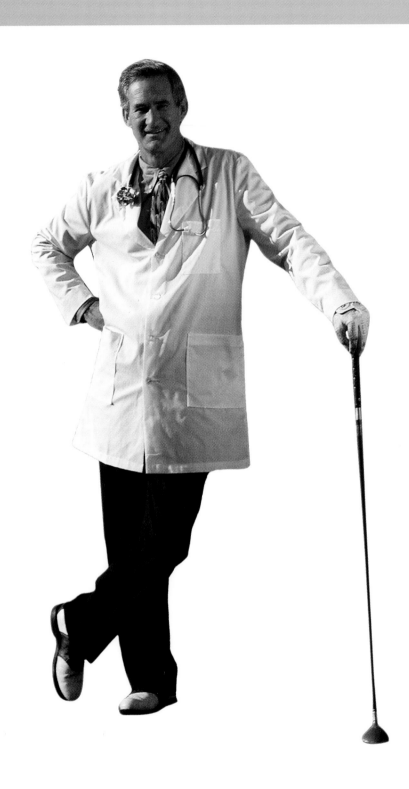

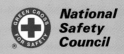
The Golf Doc

Health, Humor, and Insight to Improve Your Game

Ed Palank, MD
foreword by
Chi Chi Rodriguez

JONES AND BARTLETT PUBLISHERS
Sudbury, Massachusetts
BOSTON   TORONTO   LONDON   SINGAPORE

World Headquarters
Jones and Bartlett Publishers
40 Tall Pine Drive
Sudbury, MA 01776
978-443-5000
info@jbpub.com
www.jbpub.com

Jones and Bartlett Publishers Canada
2100 Bloor St. West
Suite 6-272
Toronto, ON M6S 5A5
CANADA

Jones and Bartlett Publishers International
Barb House, Barb Mews
London W6 7PA
UK

The first aid and CPR procedures in this book are based on the most current recommendations of responsible medical sources. The National Safety Council® and the publisher, however, make no guarantee as to, and assume no responsibility for the correctness, sufficiency or completeness of such information or recommendations. Other or additional safety measures may be required under particular circumstances.

GolfDigest® is a registered trademark of The New York Times Company Magazine Group, Inc.

Library of Congress Cataloging-in-Publication Data
Palank, Edward, 1945–
      The golf doc: health, humor, and insight to improve your game /
Edward Palank.
          p.   cm.
      Includes bibliographical references and index.
      ISBN 0-7637-1228-0
     1.   Golfers—Health and hygiene. 2. Golf injuries—Prevention.
 I. Title.
RC1220.G64P34   2000
 613'. 008'79635—dc21   99-44501
                                                              CIP

Chief Executive Officer: Clayton E. Jones
Chief Operating Officer: Don Jones, Jr.
President: Tom Walker
VP, Sales and Marketing: Tom Manning
VP, Managing Editor: Judith H. Hauck
Director of Design and Production: Anne Spencer
Director of Manufacturing and Inventory Control: Therese Bräuer
Production Editor: Rebecca S. Marks
Developmental Editor: Dean DeChambeau
Editorial/Production Assistant: Jennifer Reed
Cover and Text Design: Anne Spencer
Manufacturing Buyer: Kristen Guevara
Printing and Binding: World Color Book Services
Cover Printing: World Color Book Services

Publisher, EMS and Aquatic: Larry Newell
Associate Editor, EMS: Kathryn Twombly
Marketing Manager, EMS: Kim Brophy
Production Team: Mark Rodrigues
                  AnneMarie Lemoine
                  Stephanie Torta

Printed in the United States of America
03 02 01 00 99   10 9 8 7 6 5 4 3 2 1

To the memory of my dad,
Edward A. Palank, MD,
who showed me
the honor of being a physician.

To my mother,
Toni Palank Casey,
who, by her example, showed me
what strength is.

To my wonderful children,
Kristen and Marliese,
for their love, support, and
great sense of humor.

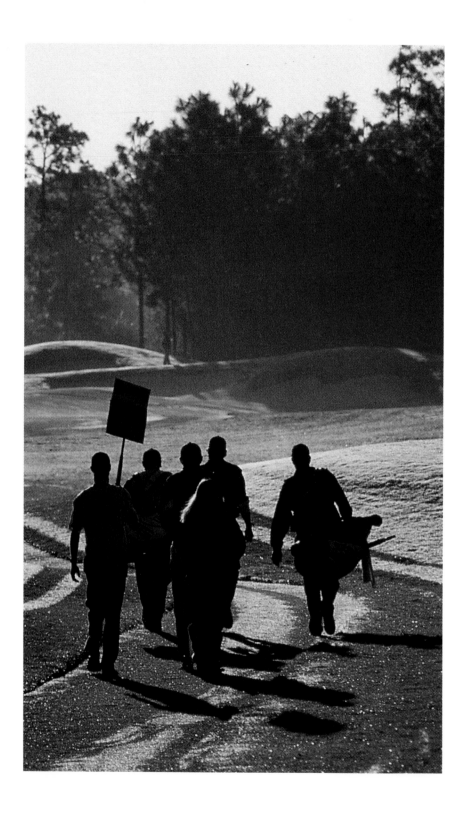

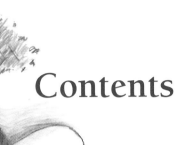

Contents

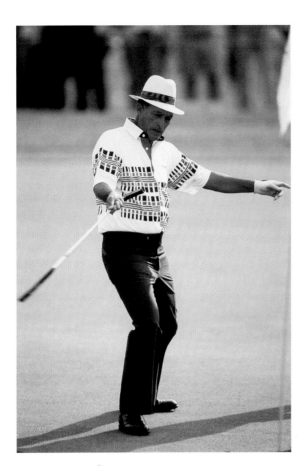

Foreword

by Chi Chi Rodriguez

It has been forty years since I became a professional golfer, and a bit longer since I learned to play in Puerto Rico with clubs made from guava tree sticks and balls fashioned from tin cans. During my professional years, I have seen technological advances in the game—balls that fly farther and clubs that hit them more accurately. I have seen gadgets of all kinds for improving the golf swing. I have witnessed players at every level eagerly try out the newest innovations, while others look to the heavens for divine intervention as they struggle to overcome the "yips."

But even with the changes in the game and the efforts to improve scores through technology, some things, you might say the most important things, have remained the same. The physical and mental benefits that you receive from playing never change. Since my heart attack and angioplasty in 1998, I have come to appreciate these benefits even more. You're never too old to play golf. You might get old enough where you won't play as well, but you're never to old to play the game. The youngest junior golfers benefit, too, from the sense of accomplishment, confidence, and self-respect that comes with hitting the ball down a big fairway and into that tiny cup.

I appreciate the opportunity that Dr. Ed Palank has given me to comment on this enjoyable and outstanding book. The title, **The Golf Doc: Health, Humor, and Insight to Improve Your Game,** speaks for itself. The game of golf, like no other sport, combines healthy elements like sunshine (in moderation) and fresh air, with an activity that strengthens the heart, lungs, muscles, and joints of the body. When played with the right mental outlook, golf can help reduce stress and improve concentration. If you watch me play, I hope you can tell that I believe keeping a sense of humor about the game is important. For me, humor helps to keep things in the proper perspective.

There are many myths and half-truths about golf and health. Golfers of all ages can benefit from the health tips that **The Golf Doc** provides. The advice in this book is a compilation of professional golf experience and professional medical training. I believe you will find it an entertaining and valuable tool to help you improve your game and your overall health. And I trust you will enjoy it as much as I do.

A Message from the Author

Golf and medicine have been twin passions of mine for almost as long as I can remember. My father was a general practitioner in the days when doctors ran their clinics in their own homes. My father saw patients downstairs. In my case at least, the household influence paid off; from the age of five, I knew I wanted to be a doctor myself. When my father died at the age of forty-six from a heart attack, cardiology became a natural choice for my specialty. It was too late for him, but maybe I could help other people avoid the risks that had brought him to such an early death.

My father comes into my early memories of golf, too, but in an odd way. When people ask me how I got started at the game, I usually mention playing with him a few times as a youngster, though never very often because "he was always so busy." That busyness, that intense commitment to work that was such a hallmark of his generation, was probably at least in part responsible for his dying so young. If I were his physician today, one of my most important prescriptions for him would be a simple one: play more golf.

Golf is a wonderful sport, beloved by those who play it, a mystery to those who don't. I have been addicted since the age of ten when I started playing with my younger brother at the small course at my family's club. I was sixteen when I hit my first hole in one, and I can still remember that soaring sense of triumph as I watched the ball fly home. To this day, I still hear that delicious swirling sound of the ball rolling into the bottom of the cup. I'd have to say now that it was sheer luck but it gave me a taste of one of the game's sweetest moments and whetted my appetite for more.

In college, I had a summer job delivering mail. A public golf course was on my route and I planned it so that I would arrive there right at my lunch hour. I would deliver the mail, play four holes, jump back in the truck, and continue the route. It was a great summer.

It was also my last intense involvement in the sport for many years. Medical school, internship, and residency left virtually no time for fun (although I did manage to get married—some things are just too important to put off!). In 1975, a full-fledged cardiologist at last, I was sent to Germany by the U.S. Army to work at a major referral center there. When I returned in 1977, I accepted an offer to set up a practice in Manchester, New Hampshire.

For the first two years, I ran my practice alone and literally never took a day off. I had two young daughters (Kristin was born in 1973 and Marliese in 1976) by then, so spare time for golf wasn't really an issue. In those days, I could barely remember how it felt to swing my clubs, let alone find them behind the strollers, diaper bags, and push toys in the closet.

In 1979 I took on a partner, the girls crossed that magic line from babyhood to childhood and suddenly life began to restructure itself into a pattern I had almost forgotten could be possible. I am still too busy with work to be anything more than a weekend golfer, but I try to make the most of it. My handicap is down to 7 and I find the challenge of the game even more exciting now than when I was young and had all the time in the world.

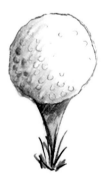

Acknowledgments

The concept for this book originated from my family and my patients. My thanks go to my brothers, Gary, Brian, and David, who make up our foursome in the annual "Palank Invitational" event. To my sister, Cynthia, whose wit keeps us all honest and grounded. My patients have been a never ending source of ideas and encouragement—together we have helped each other. My former partners and colleagues at Catholic Medical Center in Manchester, New Hampshire, helped me in medical areas where I lacked expertise.

A special thanks goes to Joe Sullivan and Jo Chopra. This book would never have been possible without the help and influence of MR to whom I am eternally grateful.

Thanks also to my playing partners at New Seabury on Cape Cod and Bay Colony in Naples; to PGA Professionals Ricky Coleman, Dean Faucher, Mike Pry, Jeff Rainer, Bruce Westemeier, Charise DeMao, Dick Dichard, and John Carroll, who were never ending sources of stories and encouragement; to Dr. Marilyn Varcoe for her help with the mental aspect of the game; and to Scott Smith and Bob Carney of *Golf Digest* for their guidance and suggestions. I would like to thank Mike Drepanos for his contribution to the Junior section of this book and his friendship to my family.

Enough thanks cannot go to Jones and Bartlett Publishers for the incredible effort in making this project a reality. The Jones and Bartlett team of Clayton Jones, Larry Newell, Dean DeChambeau, Tom Walker, Tom Manning, Anne Spencer, Rebecca Marks, Mark Rodrigues, Kim Brophy, Jennifer Reed, and Kathryn Twombly is outstanding.

Since this project took a few more years than I intended, I am especially thankful to the woman who kept me on track and typed this manuscript more times than she cares to think about, my administrative assistant, Linda Mitchell.

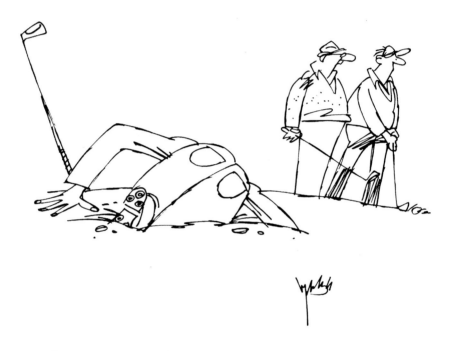

"CHARLIE JUST FELL IN YOUR DIVOT..."

Introduction

The nature of golf makes it possible for very different people at very different skill levels to play to their full potential without being frustrated by other players' abilities. Indeed, this is one of the real beauties of golf—because your true opponent is yourself, you can play with anyone, and feel neither held back nor unfairly pushed. You are the whole story.

Precisely because this is true, because the story is you and is played out with your body, it is vital that you take good care of yourself. Of course, this is true in any sport, but in golf it needs special emphasis. In most sports, good physical condition is a prerequisite for playing. It's rare to hear of someone taking up soccer, say, at the age of sixty-five, becoming passionately addicted and playing every day for the next fifteen years. In golf, it's commonplace. People routinely discover golf when they are ready to retire, at an age when physical problems are also, unfortunately, routine.

Diabetes, heart disease, and high blood pressure are all statistically more likely to affect older people, the very ones who might be spending the most time out on the golf course. The medications required for these conditions present a whole range of questions for golfers who want to play eighteen holes and still take their medication on schedule.

Although the older golfer has a higher incidence of inherent physical problems, there are other risks associated with the sport that all players should be mindful of, regardless of their age. Being in the great outdoors is one of the greatest delights of the sport, but it is also one of its hazards. Four to five hours in the sun demands defensive measures against skin cancer. Tick bites and bee stings may seem like remote possibilities, but those of us who spend a bit more time in the rough than we care to admit need to guard against potentially fatal illnesses like Lyme disease. The constant wheezing and watery eyes from allergies, suffered by an amazing twenty percent of golfers, can do more to spoil a game than any number of plugged lies or pulled shots. Lightning, which is probably the last thing most people worry about, is nonetheless a real danger on the fairway: golfers insist on carrying a lightning rod whenever they play. Good nutrition, including the prevention of dehydration, is another big issue for golfers, and more closely related to a low handicap than you might imagine. Orthopedic problems, which for a time sidelined even Jack Nicklaus, can be prevented or corrected through proper training and exercise. And stress, which the game can create or reduce, may be the single most important factor in how much you enjoy your time on the green.

The connection between golf and health was something I learned from my patients. As a cardiologist, I deal with people who have suffered the enormous trauma of a heart attack or who have had to undergo bypass surgery or other coronary procedures. Time after time, I have entered their hospital rooms prepared for "the big things in life" questions. I expect to hear "When can I go back to work, Doc?" or, at least, "Is it OK to have sex?" What I hear, however, is "How soon can I get back on the golf course?"

These patients have understood, not through academic studies or laboratory experiments but out of their own experience, just how important golf is to their physical and mental well-being. For them, full recovery means eighteen holes—anything less just isn't good enough. I know this through my own experience, but since I have a scientific background, I couldn't resist trying to quantify it. I conducted a study in 1989 which confirmed that walking the golf course can actually lower cholesterol—a finding that delighted cardiologists and heart patients across the country and reaffirmed what golfers already believed. Golf is not just another pastime or leisure activity—it is a sport with enormous health benefits.

In this book, I explain in detail how to improve your golf game by staying fit and healthy. I also cover the emergency issues most likely to affect golfers. Golf is an athletic event played outdoors. It carries with it hazards associated with rigorous physical activity. These can range from orthopedic injuries to heart attacks and cardiac arrest. Problems may include anything from insect bites to lightning strikes. You can easily learn the basic skills necessary to anticipate emergencies and to assist a golfer when a minor or major medical emergency occurs. Read it right through, even if all of the problems described do not apply to you right now; an ounce of prevention is better than a pound of cure. You can learn from the experiences of other golfers and so avoid both minor and major health problems.

Although the style adopted in **The Golf Doc** is light and easy to read, it is meant to be used as a reference book as well. But nothing can replace the importance of your own physician's diagnosis and treatment. Use this book as a general guideline, but consult your own doctor for specific advice.

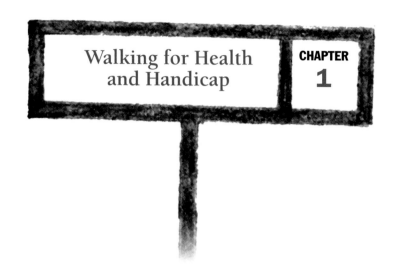

Walking for Health and Handicap

Golf combines two favorite American pastimes: taking long walks and hitting things with a stick.

— P. J. O'Rourke

I often hear my playing partners grumbling that there is no exercise involved in playing golf. Because golf is not an aerobic program in which one achieves a sustained elevated heart rate, people assume that there is little health benefit to be gained by playing this game. They're wrong! Walking the golf course will provide you with health benefits, and it will also lower your handicap.

Walk, Don't Drive, to Improve Your Health

Some time ago, I decided to try to prove scientifically that golf actually delivers both cardiovascular and vascular benefits. Many of my patients told me, time and again, that golf had proved to be their lifesaver after a heart attack, so I knew there had to be something tangible there. That many people couldn't be wrong. My study evaluated the effects walking the golf course has on cholesterol levels.[1] Players' cholesterol levels were evaluated before and after the golfing season. The study concluded that golfers who walked the course and played at least three times per week (walking twelve to fifteen miles) improved their cholesterol ratio.

The study was first published in a medical journal, but the results were picked up nationwide in the popular press. It was the news many people had been waiting for—finally, a scientific rationale for playing golf; it's indispensable for their health and well-being.

It is only by walking that we can derive the greatest physical benefits from golf. Throwing clubs doesn't count. Physicians used to advise their patients that to help their hearts at all, exercise had to be sustained and steady. We now believe that the stop-and-go pattern, which is unavoidable in golf, helps the cardiovascular system become more efficient at taking in and processing oxygen, with the overall result that one can accomplish more with less exhaustion.

If you walk the course and carry your bag, you can burn up to 380 calories per hour. As a comparison, mowing your lawn consumes 305 calories. You get more exercise golfing! In fact, according to Dr. Jim Rippe, an expert on the physiology of walking, a four-and-a-half-hour round of golf for the average male is equivalent to running two miles at a pace of eleven minutes per mile.

Calories per hour (150-pound person)

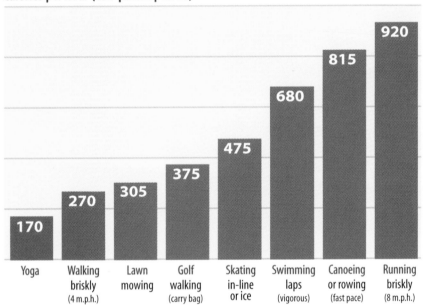

Source: *Exercise Testing and Prescription* by David Nieman; Nutrition Action HealthLetter.

Walking has other documented advantages. Engaged in regularly, it helps you to lose weight and increases muscle tone. It relieves depression and can be a substitute for addictive substances like nicotine, alcohol, and drugs. It helps cure sleep disorders and improves coordination and confidence. It will keep you young, fit, and active to the point that people many years your junior will envy you your energy.

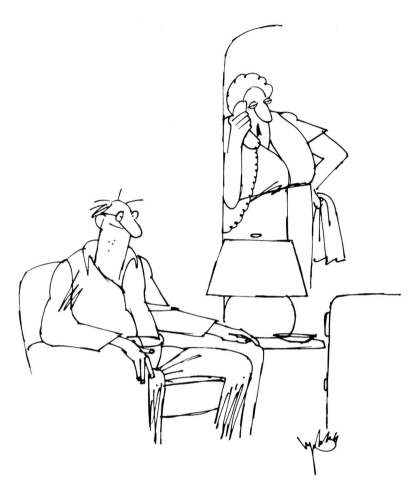

"He's tried every diet known to man. Then yesterday the doctor told him the extra weight was causing his high golf scores.... He lost 11 pounds today."

If you walk, believe it or not, you will be better equipped to deal with stress. Recognizing stress as a major risk factor in the development of heart disease marks a new phase in the medical community's understanding of the concept of cardiac well-being. Until recently, physicians tended to downplay the role of tension and emotional turmoil in the events leading up to a heart attack. Now we know better.

We also know now that one of the best strategies for reducing tension is regular, vigorous exercise. And one of the best exercises is walking.

Walking scores higher than most other exercises as a good form of fitness maintenance because it is such a natural form of movement. It requires no special equipment, no special location, and no special skills.

It can be incorporated into anyone's daily routine, practiced alone or with friends, indoors or out, and in any kind of weather.

But the greatest similarity between golf and walking is that both are lifetime pursuits. Combining these two pleasures now means that you can look forward to enjoying them until the end of your days. What more could you want?

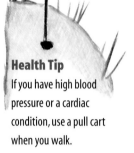

But if you still need convincing—walking is the purest way to play golf, and the game is nothing if not kept pure.

When Carts Are Necessary

You say you have difficulty walking, painful knees, or breathing problems like emphysema? Golf is a game to be enjoyed; if electric carts and motorized caddies enhance your enjoyment and minimize your pain—go for it.

Health Tip

If you have high blood pressure or a cardiac condition, use a pull cart when you walk.

Problems with carts arise in the professional golf world and the Rules of Golf as outlined by the USGA.

Many feel that walking is essential to the game. Outspoken critics, including Tom Watson and Ken Venturi, feel there should be no exceptions made to allow carts on Tour. Integral to golf is the need for players to focus and concentrate. A cart would provide an unfair advantage by minimizing fatigue and enhancing those abilities. The use of a cart also can interfere with play by matting down some of the rough, creating an unfair advantage for some players who hit an errant shot.

Casey Martin is a talented young player who has a rare circulatory disorder of his leg. He petitioned and sued the PGA Tour under the Americans with Disabilities Act for a cart to accommodate his disability that makes it painful to walk. The court ruled in favor of Martin. The Tour contends that walking is part of competitive golf and providing a cart is an unfair advantage to some players. The case is under appeal.

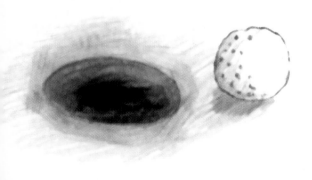

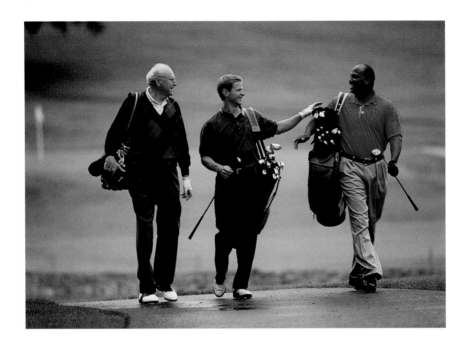

Walking to Improve Your Game

In Scotland, where golf began, there is a saying, "The game was invented a billion years ago—don't you remember?" While this may not be true, it is a certain fact that the electric golf cart is of recent vintage. Tradition, in and of itself, is not enough to determine one's decisions; but in golf its weight is a heavy one and we would do well to examine the reasons why purists scorn the idea of driving.

Golf is a game in which tempo and rhythm rule. It is hard to imagine a more perfect recipe for jagged, uneven play than the frantic activity of zipping from ball to ball in a golf cart, leaping out, flailing around with a club that has been selected with only a moment's consideration, then jumping back into the cart to speed on to the next attack. In the United States, the advent of the electric cart and its mandated use by many private clubs have virtually taken walking out of the game. Under the guise of speeding up play, some carts are even equipped with GPS (global positioning system). These sophisticated devices provide a continuous readout of the distance between the player and the green. You don't even have to walk to the sprinkler head to determine the yardage!

> *Golf is a walk in the park, not a 400-meter dash*
>
> Tom Watson

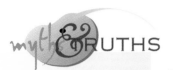

Myth: You can play more quickly with a cart.

Truth: If all of the foursome are in carts, and there is a "no cart off the path" rule in effect, your group spends as much time walking back and forth to the cart over the length of the round as you do walking directly to your ball.

Golf, as originally conceived, is a walker's game. It was developed in an easier time when people knew how to enjoy themselves, when the pleasure of the process mattered more than the end result. Having said this, however, it must also be said that in golf, as in so much else, it is the pleasure of the process that determines the end result.

Golf played skillfully provides for a graceful transition from one ball to the next, a leisurely stroll across the course with time to get a feel for the contours of the ground and to experience in one's own body the challenges and hidden facets of a particular landscape. Walking enables us to appreciate the beautiful tranquil environment and at the same time play a better game. Walking the course slows you down, no doubt about it. But golf has never been a game of speed. The relaxed pace of the game helps establish a tempo and an opportunity to analyze and to visualize the next shot. As you walk, you can prepare mentally for what lies ahead. Proper club selection can be made only after processing many variables including hazards, wind conditions, elevation, and individual abilities. When you do reach the ball, you want to be relaxed, loose, and ready to make your best shot. You are unlikely to be successful in this regard if you merely jump from cart to ball.

Every golf course is different, and, though it may sound strange, the same golf course is different every time. The course may look like one long manicured stretch, the same from one end to the other, but Nature never behaves so predictably. Unless you are able to hit your ball to exactly the same spot every time you play, the course you play today is not the same one you played yesterday or will play tomorrow. When you walk, this understanding is self-evident. Your feet know it, your eyes tell you, even your nose smells different scents as you make your way along the course. As your experience as a golfer grows, you automatically learn to incorporate your sense of geography into your game. When you drive, you lose out on the whole thing. Concentrating simply on getting from one ball to the next, you end up playing in a vacuum: it's not good golf and it's not much fun either.

Many golfers say that one of the things they like best about golf is the camaraderie, the chance to be with their friends in a beautiful setting, without contending with the usual impositions of schedules and deadlines. Walking enhances this ideal, while driving practically negates it. The very presence of a cart imposes a value of efficiency in an area where it has no place.

Links to Experience

— by Dick Dichard, PGA Professional

"Ten years ago I was playing in the Maine Open. Still in contention, I had to stop while walking up eighteen, because of tightness in my chest. The next day was worse—I had to stop five times during that round. Monday after the tournament, I told my physician about the discomfort and he recommended a stress test. Just walking on that machine gave me discomfort and instead of heading to the first tee that afternoon, I was headed to the hospital for a heart catheterization. After looking at my heart films the doctor said, 'Dick, they're not exactly even par' and recommended a balloon angioplasty. The procedure worked for a few months, but the discomfort returned. My cardiologist said because of the anatomy of my heart blood vessels (sounded something like a course layout with a high slope) that I should have a bypass.

It has now been ten years and I have never felt better. I am teaching and playing nearly every day. Walking the course has helped me lose weight and maintain my endurance. This past winter I even carried the bag for a friend who competes on the Senior Tour.

Heart surgery allowed me to return to golf. Walking has helped my game as well as my heart."

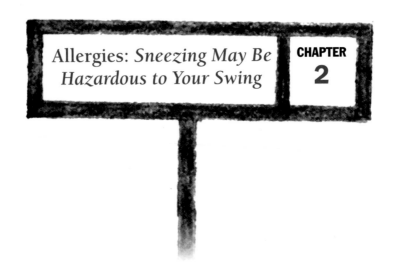

Allergies: *Sneezing May Be Hazardous to Your Swing*

CHAPTER 2

It could have been worse, I could be allergic to beer.

— Greg Norman (on his allergy to grass)

No one who suffers from allergies is happy about it, but for golfers an allergy can be a particularly cruel and unusual punishment. The perfect timing of pollen season with golf season seems to have been plotted in hell, probably by some embittered demon duffer whose handicap never went below 35 while he was on earth.

But whatever its genesis, the sad fact remains that for fifteen percent of all golfers, pollen season means trouble. Forget about bunkers and water holes—the entire golf course is a hazard. It's only logical—a well-maintained golf course is an oasis of natural beauty, ringed on all sides with trees and a variety of grasses, precisely the source of so many allergens.

What do you think about when you sit down to watch the start of the Masters' Tournament in Augusta in early spring? I know this is my chance to see some of the finest golfers in the world in action, but I can't seem to keep my mind off all that rhododendron everywhere. My eyes start to water just thinking about it. Ragweed pollen is the prime offender in the central and southern regions of the United States, with maximum pollination occurring in late August and September, just about the time when most players have begun to see the results of their summer's practice sessions on the green. While the Bermuda and bluegrasses so often found on golf courses around the country may be

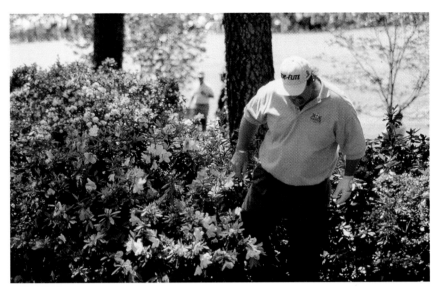

Beautiful flowers can cause some golfers trouble.

"short grass," they are still virulent allergens. The good news for allergy sufferers is that the symptoms of this affliction decrease over time. It's one situation in which a high number—your age rather than your handicap—is helpful.

Allergies are the natural response of some people's immune system to the presence of allergens like pollen, dust, and molds in the environment. All golfers, regardless of age, are susceptible to allergies. Circulating throughout the human body are mast cells, which break down whenever a susceptible individual is exposed to an allergen. In the case of an allergy to pollen, ragweed, and grasses, the mast cells break down, releasing "histamines." Histamine is a chemical that causes mucosal membranes of the nose and eyes to release fluid as a defense against the allergen. In other words, the presence of this fluid means sneezing, watery, itching eyes, runny nose, and a general feeling of discomfort. If you are an allergy sufferer, reducing your exposure to off-course irritants generated by dust, pets, and even cigarette smoke may make you less symptomatic on the course.

Help is on the way, however. If you find yourself in tears on the golf course and you are sure it's not due

Health Tip: Certain fruits may react with pollen. If you are allergic to birch pollen, you also may have symptoms if you eat apples or lemons. If you are allergic to ragweed pollen, you may have a reaction to melons.

to a botched two-foot putt for the match, a wide variety of remedies is available, ranging from over-the-counter nasal sprays, to prescription drugs, and nasal surgery.

Decongestants

Simple decongestants, available in nonprescription nasal sprays, often can provide adequate relief to many sufferers. Don't use them for more than three days, however, because they can become addictive. If you find yourself needing to use a nasal spray more frequently than recommended by the directions on the bottle, you may have developed a dependence that will have to be treated with nasal steroids. This sounds worse than it is—commonly prescribed steroids such as Nasalide® and Beconase-AQ®, will clear the congestion very quickly without the addictive side effect. You will be able to stop using them within a short time.

Health Tip
Don't wait until your sneeze affects your slice— take your medication early for best results.

When using over-the-counter medications, it's important to keep in mind other health problems you may have, as well as any other drugs you might be taking. The decongestants, for example, which act to constrict the blood vessels, may also raise your blood pressure and cause tachycardia (an abnormally rapid heartbeat). If high blood pressure is a concern, or if you have a history of cardiac disease, you'll want to consult your physician before self-prescribing. Antihistamines typically cause drowsiness, so if you are already taking sedatives for any reason, be sure that your physician is aware of this. Alcohol does not generally mix well with the antihistamines either. If the side effects of the nonprescription drugs, the most common being drowsiness, are a real problem for you, consult your physician. Often, simply switching to a different brand, or varying the dosage of your current medication will be enough to circumvent the difficulty.

Immunotherapy

If your allergy does not respond to simple measures, or if it manifests as asthma, you may want to discuss desensitization injections with your physician. This treatment program, in which allergy shots are given regularly over a three-to-four-year period, has a remarkable success rate with up to eighty percent of all patients remaining symptom free upon completion. A further fifteen percent experience some relief but cannot be considered symptom-free, even after four years of treatment.

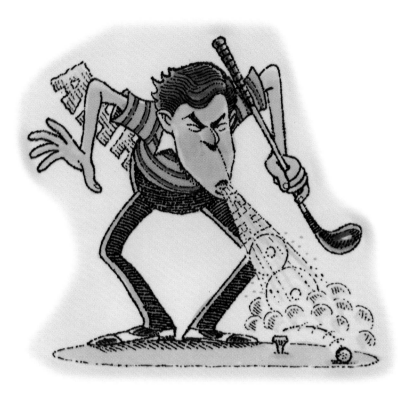

Immunotherapy, as the process is called, involves introducing into the body small quantities of the very thing to which you suffer an allergic reaction. The hope is that, over time, your own immune system will kick in and learn to fight off the unwelcome intruder. As with most invasive therapies, however, risks are involved. For approximately seven percent of people so treated, however, the immune system doesn't learn to fight—instead, they develop a systemic reaction, as if they were experiencing a full-blown allergy attack. Although there have been a small number of recorded fatalities, the risk is still extremely low considering that some ten million such injections are administered yearly.

Immunotherapy is not inexpensive, but given the fact that allergic rhinitis (inflammation of the nasal mucous membranes) is a condition that often plagues people for years on end, and factoring in the cost of some of the newer, more effective medications over that period of time, it may be the most cost-effective treatment in the long run. Sometimes a golfer just has to learn to live with this different sort of handicap. PGA Tour player

Steve Elkington has made the adjustment to a chronic allergy to grass pollen and dust. He takes two allergy injections every week and makes sure to find out which plants will be in bloom wherever he will be playing so as to arrive at a tournament well-supplied not only with his clubs and other gear but with a mini-pharmacy of anti-allergy medication as well. During the second round of the 1999 British Open in Carnoustie, Scotland, Jesper Parnevik required medical treatment for an acute episode of hay fever. He was able to obtain relief from his symptoms, and continued his round, finishing with the second best round of the day.

ALLERGIES: WHAT YOU SHOULD KNOW

WHAT TO LOOK FOR

- Recurrent bouts of repetitive sneezing
- Nasal congestion
- Itchy, watering eyes
- Runny nose
- Dry cough
- Hoarseness
- Difficulty breathing/drawing a breath
- Flushed, itchy, or burning skin
- Hives
- Swelling

WHAT TO DO

- Pollen thrives in hot, dry, windy conditions especially in the early morning. Whenever possible, play your game when it is cool, humid, and less windy.
- If pollen counts are high, consider taking an antihistamine before you play.
- Avoid allergic substances and reduce your exposure to pollen. This might mean putting off mowing your lawn—you do what have to do!

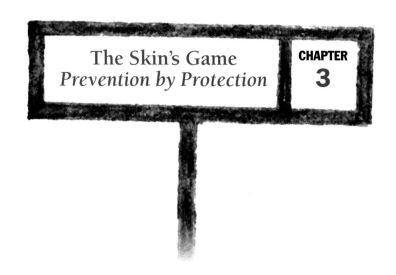

The Skin's Game
Prevention by Protection

CHAPTER 3

Never bet with anyone you meet on the first tee who has a deep suntan, a 1-iron in his bag, and squinty eyes.

—Dave Marr

We all know about the dangers of skin cancer and yet seventy percent of us (according to the National Cancer Institute and the Centers for Disease Control and Prevention) continue to ignore the experts' warnings. The market is flooded with sunscreens containing higher and higher protection factors, and the popular press is full of timely, common-sense advice on how to avoid UVA and UVB rays. Yet we go on as if we were blissfully unaware of the potential damage of being out in the sun.

There is a complicated psychological hurdle to cross before we can begin to see the sun as an adversary. Fresh air and sunshine, both of which golf provides in abundance, traditionally have been associated not with danger but with precisely its opposites: good health and well-being. Many senior golfers have retired to Arizona or Florida precisely for those states' year-round sunny climate. If the sun is shining, we automatically feel good. Depression and mental illness tend to occur in those areas where the sun shines much less often. In fact, people who work in buildings devoid of natural light are likely to get disoriented and do not perform at par. We need the sun. This need is built into our genes.

Unfortunately, many of us also have genes that simply cannot withstand the intensity of the sun that our bodies crave. Those of us with fair skin are at risk every time we go out in the sun.

The skin is the body's largest organ. It is the protective covering for every other organ, providing a suit of armor against harmful bacterial invasion. It regulates the body's temperature and guards against dehydration. It deserves, and indeed requires, at least a small amount of care; most of us, however, prefer to take its health for granted.

Cases of skin cancer have been on the increase for years now and the numbers show no sign of decreasing anytime soon. If present trends continue, more than half a million new skin cancers will occur next year in the United States alone. According to the American Cancer Society, one million new cases of nonmalignant melanoma and 44,200 new cases of melanoma will be diagnosed in 1999. Skin cancer is the most common cancer in the United States today, taking 9,200 lives in 1998 alone.

It isn't just that many people are spending more time in the sun. The sad fact is that exposure to the

myth & TRUTHS

Myth: Sunscreen is sufficient protection against the common forms of skin cancer. **Truth:** Unfortunately, sunscreens may not fully protect against the deadly skin cancer melanoma. Wide-brimmed hats and tight-knit clothing should be used for protection as well.

Years of sun damage have taken its toll on the skin of this beach community resident. The photo on the left was taken with a standard camera lens. The photo on the right was taken with an ultraviolet camera lens and shows the damage under the surface of the skin.

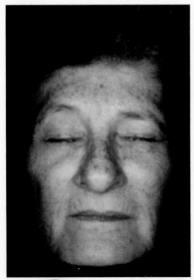 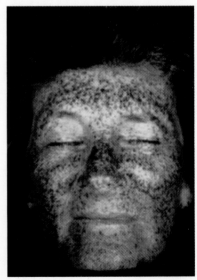

Source: (AAD) *Courtesy of the American Academy of Dermatologists (AAD).*

sun at all is more dangerous than it used to be. Chlorofluorocarbons, the chemicals found in aerosols and refrigerants, have been depleting the ozone layer of the earth's stratosphere at a rate rapid enough to cause grave concern. The diminishment of the ozone layer allows more and more harmful ultraviolet radiation to reach the earth. There is a strange justice in the process: as we destroy the earth's protective "skin," our own skin suffers too.

United States Open champion Andy North thought he had been careful about his exposure to both UVA and UVB rays, applying sunscreen for the past fifteen years. But as he points out, and oncologists agree with

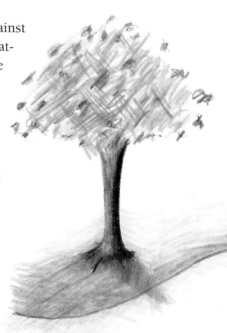

Health Tip

A polo shirt has an SPF of only 8, and if wet, an SPF of 6.

him, for most people, the sun damage is done long before it starts showing on the skin. Skin cancer is a cumulative disease—the sunbathing you did as a teenager will only come back to haunt you when you are in your forties. And in any case, what forty-year-old even had heard of sunscreens in his or her teens? Andy North's cancer appeared on his face, and was serious enough to require five operations and eventually plastic surgery.

Obviously you can't rewrite history. If you spent your share of time at the beach as a reckless teenager, there's nothing you can do about it now.

All it takes is six bad sunburns in your past to increase your risk of developing skin cancer today by two and a half times. It's never too late to protect your skin. What you can do now is minimize further damage and make sure that your children and grandchildren don't make the same mistakes you did.

The strategies for protecting yourself against the sun may seem time-consuming and irritating in the beginning, but once you incorporate them into your daily golf routine, they will become second nature: soon you will no more think of heading to the course without sunscreen than you would without your clubs.

First, don't even think of playing golf until you have applied sunscreen. Slather it on wherever skin is exposed—don't forget odd spots like the tops of your ears and the back of your neck. Use a lip protection stick liberally, whenever possible. Second, avoid playing when the sun is at its peak between 11:00 A.M. and 3:00 P.M. Schedule your tee time for early morning or late afternoon. Keep in mind that your geographic location makes a big difference in the intensity of UV radiation. If you play in Florida, for example, you get one and a half times more UV rays than your counterpart in the Northeast. High altitudes also mean higher doses: for every 1,000 feet you climb above sea level, your UV exposure increases by four percent. Finally, when you are playing a course with a lot of water or white sand, be aware that the sun's rays are more intense when they are reflected.

Look for the phrase "broad spectrum" on the sunscreen bottle. In order to be completely protected, the skin needs a barrier from both UVA and UVB rays. Look for sunscreen containing Parsol 1789. This ingredient has the ability to block both UVA and UVB rays.

Which sunscreen you use depends entirely upon you and your personal preference. Today an enormous range is available for you to choose from—there are creams, sprays, gels, roll-ons, and even sunscreen towelettes. Many products are nongreasy, so that applying them need not cause a slippery grip. Both sprays and roll-ons practically eliminate this problem in any case. For those with dry skin, a cream-based sunscreen will provide skin with both protection and moisture. For oilier complexions, a gel-based sunscreen will provide protection without a greasy feel. For those golfers with sensitive skin, there are hypoallergenic and noncomedogenic versions on the market.

"Sweat-resistant" sunscreen will keep on working for thirty minutes on people who perspire heavily. A "water-resistant" product will protect for eighty minutes in the water. These numbers are important to keep in mind. Sunscreen is not a magic ointment you can put on once and then forget about. Like almost everything else in life, it needs maintenance.

Health Tip

Certain drugs increase your sensitivity to the sun and are known as phototoxic or photosensitive

- **Antibiotics:** sulfonamides, tetracyclines, trimethoprin
- **Topical steroids:** hydrocortisone
- **Nonsteroidal anti-inflammatories (NSAIDs):** aspirin, ibuprofen, naproxen
- **Tranquilizers:** benzodiazepines, tricyclics
- **Cardiac medications:** amiodarone, diltiazem, nifedipine
- **Diuretics:** thiazides, furosemide (lasix)
- **Retinoids:** Retina A
- **Diabetic medication:** sulfonylurea (orinase)

The other number you need to be aware of is the SPF of your sunscreen. What is SPF? Sun Protective Factor (SPF) is a relative number which tells you how long you can stay in the sun safely. For example, if you have very fair skin and you start to burn within twenty minutes of going out in the sun, sunscreen with an SPF of 15 will allow you to stay out fifteen times longer without burning. That's five hours, about the time most people take to play eighteen holes on today's crowded courses. But remember that if you sweat a great deal (especially if you towel off frequently) you'll need to reapply it at least at the turn. Remember, too, to apply sunscreen at least half an hour before you intend to play—the product needs time to work effectively.

Health Tip

Use a sunscreen that is broad spectrum, that is, it blocks both UVA and UVB rays. Ultraviolet radiation is composed of UVC rays, which are completely absorbed by the ozone layer, UVA rays and UVB. The harmful rays are UVB, which damage unprotected skin, causing aging of the skin and skin cancer. The UVA rays are associated with the photosensitive and photoallergic reactions.

Links to Experience

Mark Lye

Mark Lye, a PGA Tour professional, also had a scare with skin cancer. The mole he'd been ignoring on his leg for years suddenly seemed to double in size from one week to the next. He was diagnosed days later with an aggressive malignant melanoma—the dreaded black mole skin cancer, a virulent disease which claims thousands of lives in the United States every year. Lye was lucky, though. His cancer was caught early enough that even chemotherapy was deemed unnecessary. You can bet that it changed his life, however, putting everything in a radically different perspective. "It scared the hell out of me," he says. "My drive to succeed probably isn't the same as it used to be...the three-footers really don't mean so much anymore."

Dress for Protection

Clothing is another consideration. If it's not too hot, wear a long-sleeved shirt and pants. Tight-knit, dark fabrics are the most effective against both UVA and UVB rays. White, loose-knit shirts, especially if they are wet with perspiration, may allow up to thirty percent of UV light to reach your skin. Special clothing with high UV protection can now be purchased in sport specialty stores. Solumbra is one manufacturer of lightweight clothing with an SPF of 30—effectively blocking ninety-seven percent of UVA and UVB rays.

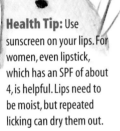

Wear a Hat

Health Tip: Use sunscreen on your lips. For women, even lipstick, which has an SPF of about 4, is helpful. Lips need to be moist, but repeated licking can dry them out.

Don't use a visor—all you will protect is your face. Go for a broad-brimmed hat that will shade the back of your neck and the top of your head as well. The hat brim should be at least three inches wide. Experts recommend wearing a four-inch wide broad-brimmed hat—one that will shade your face, ears, and the back of your neck. Avoid loosely woven straw hats. They may be stylish, but they aren't the most effective at protecting your face from the sun.

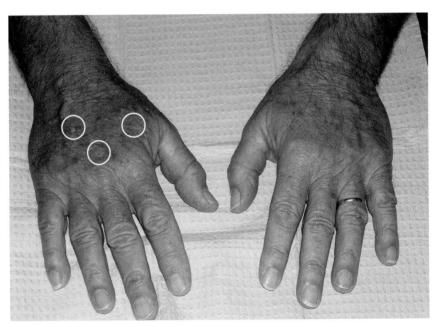

Skin damage on a golfer's nongloved hand

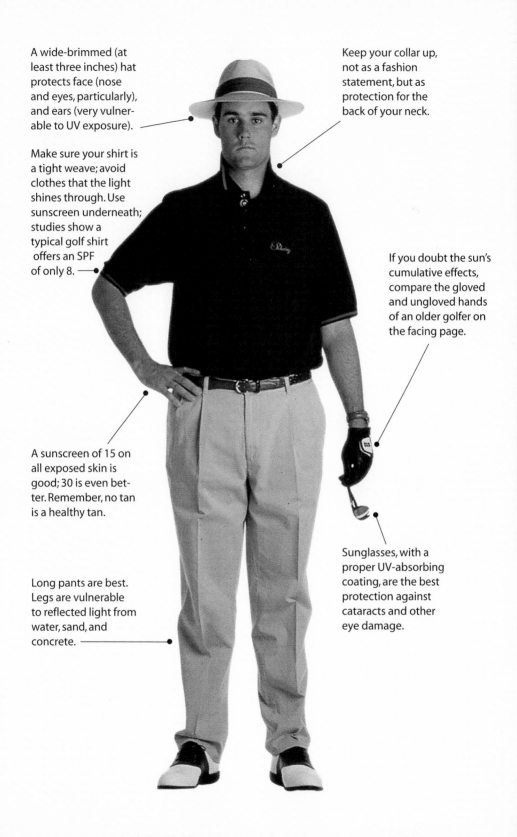

A wide-brimmed (at least three inches) hat protects face (nose and eyes, particularly), and ears (very vulnerable to UV exposure).

Make sure your shirt is a tight weave; avoid clothes that the light shines through. Use sunscreen underneath; studies show a typical golf shirt offers an SPF of only 8.

Keep your collar up, not as a fashion statement, but as protection for the back of your neck.

If you doubt the sun's cumulative effects, compare the gloved and ungloved hands of an older golfer on the facing page.

A sunscreen of 15 on all exposed skin is good; 30 is even better. Remember, no tan is a healthy tan.

Long pants are best. Legs are vulnerable to reflected light from water, sand, and concrete.

Sunglasses, with a proper UV-absorbing coating, are the best protection against cataracts and other eye damage.

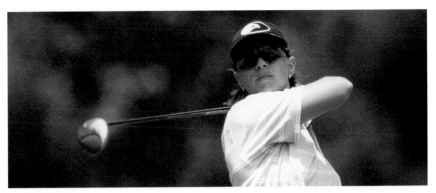

Annika Sorenstam

Use Protective Eyewear

Remember to protect your eyes with sunglasses. The evidence is clear that UV rays cause both cataracts and macular degeneration. Cataracts can be cured with surgery (although it's not exactly a pleasant procedure), but macular degeneration—in which one's central vision disappears entirely—can seldom be reversed. When choosing sunglasses, therefore, be very sure that the ones you buy protect from UV rays. Sunglasses with UV protection always carry a sticker stating such on the lenses. Wrap-around sunglasses with ninety percent or higher UV absorption offer the most protection. Many people do their eyes more harm than good by wearing sunglasses that have little or no UV protection. The retina opens up wide in the darkness and more UV rays get in than would have had the person worn no sunglasses at all.

Check Yourself

Finally, check your skin periodically. Use a full-length mirror or ask a friend or family member to check hard-to-see areas like the back of your neck, behind your ears, and your back. No matter how long you've been going to the same physician, he or she will never know your body as well as you do. Some golfers are more at risk for sun damage and aging of the skin; they include golfers who have fair skin or freckles, tend to burn easily, or have a family history of skin cancer. Pay attention to moles and dark spots, regardless of their size. Check with your physician immediately if a mole suddenly changes in size or color, or if it bleeds, becomes itchy, or changes in any other way. Do not delay. Most skin cancers are 100 percent curable if they are caught in the earliest stages. If your mole is determined to be cancerous or even precancerous, it will probably be removed in a minor surgery and you will be able to return home the same day. There usually will be a small scar—a small price to pay.

PREVENTION: WHAT YOU SHOULD KNOW

WHAT TO DO

- Use sunscreen and lip balm with an SPF of at least 15.
- Use sunscreen on cloudy days.
- Apply sunscreen at least thirty minutes before going out in the sun.
- Don't forget to put sunscreen on your ears.
- Avoid peak sun time between 11:00 A.M. and 3:00 P.M.
- Wear a hat and sunglasses with UVA/UVB protection.
- Examine your skin regularly for irregularities and changes.

WHAT TO LOOK FOR

The ABCD rule is a useful tool to check for signs of melanoma. See your physician if you see any of the following changes to your mole or birthmark:

- A is for ASYMMETRY: One-half of a mole or birthmark does not match the other.
- B is for BORDER: The edges are irregular, ragged, notched, or blurred.
- C is for COLOR: The color is not the same all over, but may have differing shades of brown or black, sometimes with patches of red, white, or blue.
- D is for DIAMETER: The area is larger than six millimeters (about the size of a pencil eraser) or is growing larger.

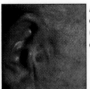 Actinic eratoses (precancerous lesion)

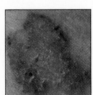 Basal cell carcinoma

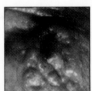 Squamous cell carcinoma

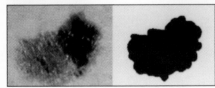

Assymetry—one half unlike the other half

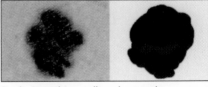

Border irregular—scalloped or poorly circumscribed border

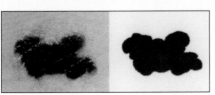

Color varied from one area to another; shades of tan and brown; black; sometimes white, red or blue

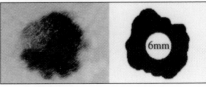

Diameter larger than six millimeters as a rule (diameter of a pencil eraser)

Source: *Courtesy of the American Academy of Dermatologists (AAD).*

Poison Ivy, Oak, and Sumac

In addition to your skin being assaulted by the sun, any contact with poisonous vegetation may result in a reaction characterized by redness and swelling. The most likely culprits for the golfer are poison ivy, poison oak, and poison sumac. Poison ivy can be found in every U.S. state except Hawaii and Alaska. The two types of poison oak are Western and Southern. Sumac is found in the swamps of the East and South. If you're one of the fifty percent of golfers who is sensitive to the plant's resin, touching these plants will result in a rash. Within eight and forty-eight hours, a line of small blisters will appear where your skin touched the plant, followed by redness and swelling with larger blisters, and severe itching. The reaction usually takes twelve days to run its course.

myth & TRUTHS

Myth: You can get poison ivy from touching someone's rash.
Truth: The reaction caused by poison ivy is not contagious. The blister fluid does not contain the irritant.

Prevention is the best way to treat potentially harmful greenery. Learn to recognize these plants. If you're hosting out-of-town guests and your home course has these plants, make sure your guests know how to recognize them. Keep a sharp eye out for poisonous plants when looking for your ball in the rough. It's not wise to retrieve a ball from the middle of a poison ivy patch.

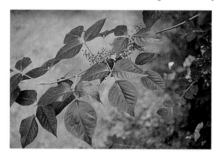

Poison ivy

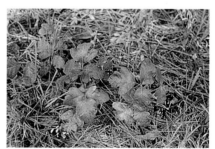

Poison oak

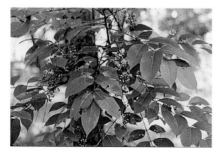

Poison sumac

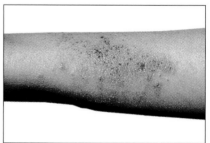

Poison ivy dermatitis

CONTACT WITH POISONOUS PLANTS: WHAT YOU SHOULD KNOW

WHAT TO LOOK FOR

- A raised red rash
- Itching and mild swelling that occurs within eight hours of contact
- A distinct line of small blisters
- A reaction that generally lasts for twelve days

WHAT TO DO

- Wash with cold running water as quickly as possible after the known contact. The resin in the plants is firmly fixed to the skin within thirty minutes.
- Avoid scratching. You can spread the resin to other parts of your body soon after contact.
- Take cool baths and apply cold, wet packs to reduce itching.
- Apply calamine lotion or hydrocortisone ointment.
- For more severe, large-scale rashes, seek medical care.
- Apply antihistamines and lotions that may provide relief from itching, but do not alter the course of the eruption.

Contact Dermatitis from Your Glove

Chemicals and even certain soaps may result in inflammation to the area of contact. If you notice a reaction just on your left hand that is similar to poison ivy, it may be a reaction to the chemicals in your golf glove. For left-handed golfers, the right hand will be affected. Treatment is similar to that for poison ivy. In addition, using a glove made of a different material can help.

SKIN REACTIONS: WHAT YOU SHOULD KNOW

WHAT TO LOOK FOR

- Red rash only on the gloved hand

WHAT TO DO

- Switch to a glove of a different material.
- Apply hydrocortisone cream to the affected area.

Acne on Your Upper Leg?
It's Your Tee!

As if your skin isn't taking enough abuse from the effects of the sun, poison ivy, and pesticides, consider what damage tees can do to your skin.

Most of us carry our used tees in our front pants pockets. As we make our swing with that beautiful full body turn, the tees tucked away in a pocket occasionally perforate the lining and make a small puncture in the skin of the upper leg. We are in essence inoculating our skin with bacteria introduced from that recently used and now contaminated tee. The result is a small area of pimples or pustules on the upper thigh adjacent to the pocket.

LEG ACNE: WHAT YOU SHOULD KNOW

WHAT TO LOOK FOR

- Presence of red raised pimples or pustule on upper thigh in region of pants pocket

WHAT TO DO

- Keep your tees elsewhere.
- The eruption will generally resolve on its own and not require specific treatment.
- If the infection persists, antibiotics may be required. See your physician.

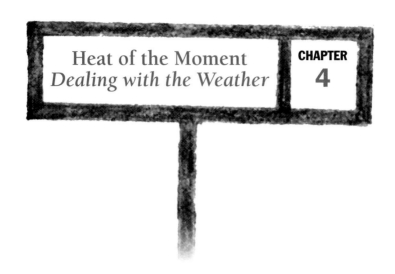

Heat of the Moment
Dealing with the Weather

CHAPTER 4

I play in the low 80s. If it's any hotter than that, I won't play.

—Joe E. Lewis

The year 1964: The U.S. Open at Washington, D.C., with Ken Venturi a strong contender for the championship. He had surprised many people by being there at all. Although his performance in the fifties was so outstanding he was often compared favorably to Ben Hogan, by 1960 something clearly had gone wrong. His game deteriorated and his marriage and health also suffered. He continued to play, but a series of minor injuries made it more and more difficult. The magic was gone.

By 1963 his belief in himself was faltering and he was seen as a has-been. Companies were no longer approaching him for endorsements, and he was teetering on the edge of bankruptcy. But in 1964, with the sympathetic support of his parish priest, Venturi somehow found the strength to begin rebuilding his life. Although he did not actually win a tournament, his game improved dramatically, and he was able to qualify for the U.S. Open.

The weather that year was unbelievably hot, even for Washington: 100°F with humidity at ninety percent. I was eighteen at the time and I had been in the gallery on the second-to-last day. I remember the stillness of the air and the way the raised clubs seemed to shimmer in the heat. Those of us watching could stand under the trees, but for the players out on the open fairway, the sun must have been brutal. I missed the chance to attend on the dramatic last day, but I consoled myself by saying it was just too hot to be outside. What I missed, however, made golfing history.

On the last day of the U.S. Open, tradition required that thirty-six, not eighteen, holes be played. Early in the morning, Ken Venturi took over the lead, playing his best game in years. As the day wore on, however, the heat began to take its toll. Lightheaded and dehydrated, he finally collapsed in the clubhouse and had to be revived with intravenous fluids. The physician attending him told him in no uncertain terms that he should not continue playing, but Venturi's mind was made up. Victory was so close he could taste it—it was a victory he needed not only as a professional, but as a human being.

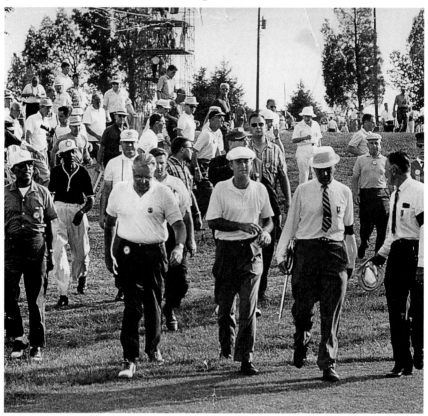

Ken Venturi (center) at the 1964 U.S. Open at Oakmont

Both his doctor and his friend, the priest, hovered anxiously beside him as he practically lurched through the last few holes. USGA Executive Director, Joe Dey, was so moved by the sight of the valiant player that he brushed aside Venturi's willingness to be penalized for his exceptionally slow progress. "Just hold your chin up proudly and keep walking," Dey told him. "You're about to be the U.S. Open champion."

Dey was right. Venturi's fifteen-foot par putt on the last green was all he needed to win. As the truth dawned on him that he was indeed the champion, Venturi, already weak and exhausted from heat stroke, broke down and wept with joy and relief. He wasn't the only one. Even the player paired with him that day, a rookie by the name of Ray Floyd, was moved to tears, and few who witnessed the day's events will ever forget them. I wasn't even there, but the scene remains vividly etched in my mind. By the time I tell this tale to my grandchildren, I'll probably have myself acting as Venturi's caddie!

The upshot of it all, as far as golfers went, was also dramatic: the USGA, in an abrupt move, changed the rules of the event to allow only eighteen holes per day. Although Venturi's was an extreme case of heat exhaustion, milder versions are not uncommon. Golf is, after all, an athletic event of fairly long duration. It is typically played in the summer, often in hot climates. If we are to be successful at golf, we must know how to deal sensibly with varying weather conditions—this is true both physically and mentally.

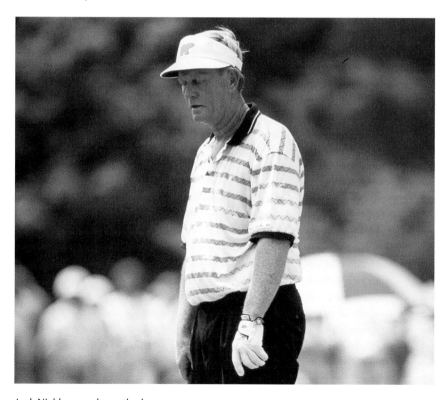

Jack Nicklaus endures the heat.

Preventing Heat Exhaustion

Heat exhaustion is easy to prevent. If you play in a hot, humid environment, take precautions. Adequate fluid intake is your number one priority. Playing in the heat means you will sweat—and when you sweat, you lose vital fluids. Start your round with a long cool drink of water and continue sipping as you play. Water is the drink of choice. Commercial sports drinks designed to replace electrolytes such as potassium and sodium are not necessary, although studies have shown that during vigorous exercise in the hot sun, a sports drink that contains glucose polymers will provide a higher fluid volume than just plain water. For most golfers, however, this amounts to overkill.

Health Tip
Cold water will cool you better than water at room temperature. Carry water with you in an insulated drinking bottle or wrap a bottle in a wet towel. You can use the wet towel to wipe your face and neck.

Avoid alcoholic drinks and anything that contains caffeine. That cold beer, cola, or iced coffee has a diuretic effect (meaning increased urination) and may turn a mild case of dehydration into something more serious. Caffeine also causes the jitters in many people, making that crucial three-foot putt even more difficult. It's well known that alcohol slows down responses and causes a general decline in performance, but alcohol also can enhance susceptibility to heat stroke.

Remember that thirst is not a reliable indicator of the body's need for water. Regular pauses at the water fountain should become part of your golfing routine. Don't wait for your body to demand water: by then it becomes difficult to replenish the fluids you have lost. In hot weather, a golfer can lose up to two quarts of sweat per hour.

The 1999 PGA Western Open was played in July outside of Chicago on a day when the temperature was in the nineties with high humidity. Garland Dempsey was the fifty-one-year-old caddie for professional golfer John Maginnes. While walking down the fifteenth fairway, Dempsey collapsed. Maginnes and Matt Moore, a spotter for ABC television, immediately started CPR. Paramedics used an automatic external defibrillator (AED) to restart his heart while he was lying on the fairway. After they restored his heart rhythm and gave him IV fluids, he was stabilized and taken to the hospital.

A caddie also collapsed during the previous year's Western Open. Greg Kraft's caddie suffered from heatstroke during the third round, but recovered after being given IV fluids. As a result of the incident at the 1999 Western

Open, the PGA ruled that on days when the heat index exceeds 100 degrees, caddies may wear short pants (see p. 30).

Take the time to let your body acclimatize to the heat. This is especially necessary for golfers who flee to warmer climates in the winter. If you have been battling winter winds in Vermont and suddenly find yourself transported to Arizona or Florida, you're going to need time to adjust. You'll be vulnerable to heat illness, so don't ruin your game by overdoing it in the first few days. Take it slowly, playing primarily in the cooler morning or evening hours until your body is ready for total luxury!

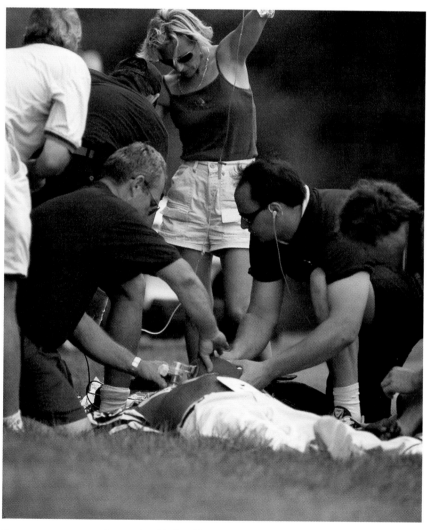

Emergency personnel attend to Garland Dempsey at the 1999 Western Open.

Pay attention to the way you dress, choosing fabrics that "breathe," such as cotton. Don't forget to wear a hat or, at the very least, a visor. On severely hot days, consider taking short breaks under the trees. Salt tablets are unnecessary and dangerous—your body retains liquid when you take them, but the liquid gets stored in the blood vessels, not in the tissues where it is needed.

Certain medications also interfere with the body's natural ability to cope with extreme heat. Heart medicines, such as beta blockers and calcium blockers, decrease your body's ability to respond to heat stress—they limit blood flow to the skin. Ask your physician about your particular prescription. Decongestants tend to constrict blood vessels, so they also limit the flow of blood to the skin. Antihistamines, tranquilizers, and antidepressants inhibit sweat gland function, thereby increasing the risk of heat stroke. People on diuretics may want to consider taking their medication after their round to avoid the potential problem of dehydration, at least on very hot, humid days.

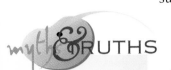

Myth: Taking salt tablets before the round and chugging a commercial sport drink during the round combat possible dehydration.
Truth: Taking salt tablets is harmful and should be avoided. Concern for adequate fluid replacement is commendable, but water is fine, and there is no need for commercial sport drinks. If you are thirsty while playing, you are already behind in your fluids.

Heat Index

Relative Humidity, %	Air Temperature, °F										
	70	75	80	85	90	95	100	105	110	115	120
	Apparent Temperature, °F										
0	64	69	73	78	83	87	91	95	99	103	107
10	65	70	75	80	85	90	95	100	105	111	116
20	66	72	77	82	87	93	99	105	112	120	130
30	67	73	78	84	90	96	104	113	123	135	148
40	68	74	79	86	93	101	110	123	137	151	
50	69	75	81	88	96	107	120	135	150		
60	70	76	82	90	100	114	132	149			
70	70	77	85	93	106	124	144				
80	71	78	86	97	113	136					
90	71	79	88	102	122						
100	72	80	91	108							

Above 130°F = heatstroke imminent
105°–130°F = heat exhaustion and heat cramps likely; heatstroke with long exposure and activity
90°–105°F = heat exhaustion and heat cramps with long exposure and activity
80°–90°F = fatigue during exposure and activity

Source: National Weather Service.

PLAYING GOLF IN THE HEAT: WHAT YOU SHOULD KNOW

- Both walking and carrying your bag will increase the body's heat production, so pace yourself accordingly.
- When humidity exceeds seventy-five percent, heat evaporation from the body essentially stops.
- Water is the best replacement fluid. Cold water will not cause cramps.
- Salt tablets are dangerous and should be avoided.
- Alcohol may exacerbate dehydration and should not be used for fluid replacement.

Wind and Rain

For most of us, four to five hours free and clear are not that easy to come by. We look forward to our time on the golf course all week—unless there's a real downpour and a hurricane watch is in effect, we mean to get out there and play. Our friends in Scotland and England have to deal with rain on an almost daily basis—if they can manage it, why can't we?

All the same, adequate protection from the elements will make a big difference in how much we actually enjoy the experience. There is little point in marching bravely through eighteen holes, soaked to the skin, shivering with cold but full of grim determination. Remember, golf is supposed to be fun!

Golf is, first of all, a game of concentration. To really focus on the ball and where we want it to go, we need to be free of distractions. Little nagging discomforts, such as cold feet or wet clothes, can become so irritating that we forget why we are really there. Taking care of the small details makes it possible for us to attend to the game.

Health Tip: A golfer exposed to a summer hailstorm while wearing only a t-shirt and shorts is more likely to become hypothermic than a well-dressed skier in the winter. Carry a jacket or sweater in your bag.

Comfort is closely related to heat. If the weather is chilly, your body will lose heat. If, in addition, your clothes are damp with perspiration or actually wet due to rain or mist, you will lose heat even faster—up to twenty-three times as fast! (See Chapter 21 for signs of hypothermia.) It is important, therefore, to choose protective clothing carefully.

There is so much available on the market today, however, that making that choice has become rather difficult! Miracle fabrics abound with each one promising (and many actually delivering!) an array of benefits about which golfers of twenty years ago could only dream. Tammie Green, an LPGA professional, noted that "a quality fabric extends my season, adding months of pleasure to each year."

Every individual's choice of clothing will vary according to the climate in which he or she plays and the limits to which one pushes the golf season. For some people, water-resistant fabric will be adequate, while others (those planning to play in the Pebble Beach Pro Am, for example) will need something actually water-proof. Since we sweat, our body produces a natural moisture vapor. It is important that our clothing allows transmission of the vapor to the outside. "Breathability" of the garment is essential to our comfort. GORE-TEX® is a good choice for both warmth and dryness, but not everyone needs warmth. Proper fit is essential: make sure when the jacket is fully zipped that there are no restrictions to the arms or back that might interfere with your swing.

Choose your clothing as you would your clubs. I won't go so far as to say that they are as important to your game, but they are certainly a close second.

PLAYING IN THE COLD OR RAIN: WHAT YOU SHOULD KNOW

WHAT TO DO

- A good overall strategy is to dress in layers that you can peel off as you warm up and add back on as you cool down.
- Wear a warm hat. Much of your body heat escapes through your head.
- Carry an extra pair of socks in case your feet get soaked.
- Choose hats with brims which help keep the water from dripping off your nose as you're trying to putt in the rain.

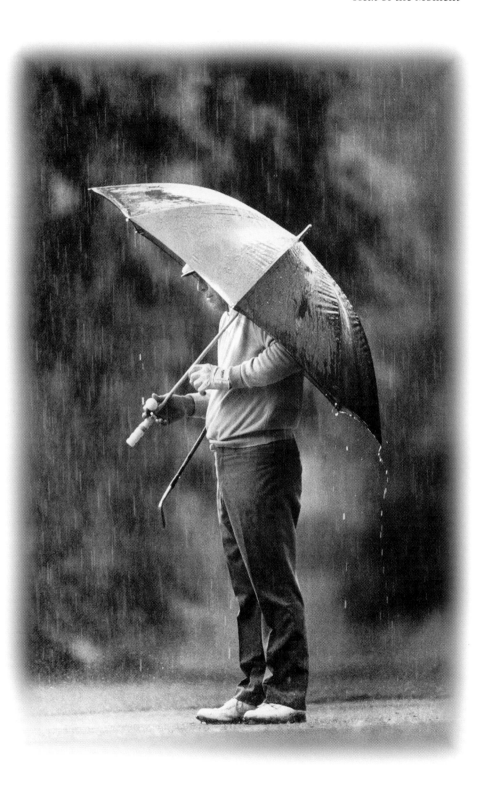

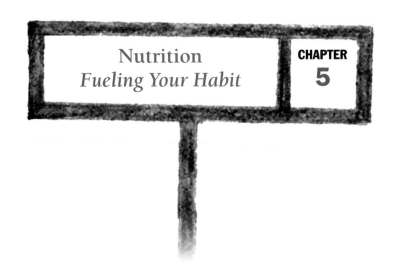

Nutrition
Fueling Your Habit

CHAPTER 5

One of the nice things about the Senior Tour is that we can take a cart and cooler. If your game is not going well, you can always have a picnic.

—Lee Trevino

If you are making your morning donut dash before heading for the course or looking for the golden arches at the turn, don't expect to shoot your career round. You can't cut the dogleg on nutrition. Athletes in any sport will tell you that diet plays an important role in their performance. Golf is an activity of moderate intensity but long duration. It is important to supply your muscles with adequate fuel, found in carbohydrates, in order to avoid fatigue and exhaustion. The dietary needs of the golfer are not much different from those other athletes.

If you skip breakfast because of your early tee time, you will find that you will be tired and hungry during the entire round. Before heading to the course, consider eating cereal, toast, bagels, or English muffins, but go light on the butter and high-fat spreads. Try jam instead, or honey. Muffins and donuts with high fat content will take longer to digest and will impair your performance. Try eating one to two hours before playing, which allows time for digestion.

Eating adequate calories from different foods will satisfy your need for carbohydrates, protein, fat, and vitamins. A diet high in carbohydrates increases glycogen stores, your source of energy. Seventy percent of the calories you consume daily should come from carbohydrates in the form of bread, cereals, pasta, vegetables, and fruit. Fat is an important energy source for those activities that are prolonged and low in intensity. Protein plays only a small role in energy production.

Vitamins and Nutritional Supplements

Today there is much talk about nutritional supplements and the use of vitamins. Given the size of the vitamin aisle at the local pharmacy, we should be the healthiest people in the world. Pills of every size, shape, and color, in capsules, tablets, and chewables line the shelves. Talk about confusion! Should we take them? Which ones are the best? Chromium, tryptophan, and carnitine are not only difficult to pronounce but they sound more like ingredients for a bomb than elements to make us healthier.

myth & TRUTHS

Myth: Vitamins provide energy.
Truth: There is no evidence that vitamins enhance athletic performance or provide energy if taken in megadoses.

Vitamins are food substances that assist in chemical reactions in your body. The best source of vitamins comes from a diet containing a variety of wholesome foods. The recommended daily allowance (RDA) can be met with an adequate diet. Choose foods that are natural powerhouses. Fruits and vegetables are a great natural vitamin source and also provide fiber and other compounds that pills don't.

Creatine is an amino acid thought to enhance muscular performance. It has been advocated by baseball and football players as a strength enhancer. There is some suggestion that high-intensity performance may be improved as a result. However, unless your goal is to hit thousands of balls at the range in a short period of time, it's unlikely to help your golf game.

Chromium is a trace metal found in mushrooms, prunes, whole-grain breads, and cereals. In theory, chromium improves the use of sugar and absorption of amino acids in muscles. There is no data to suggest that it results in a leaner body mass or improved strength. In fact, increased dosages of chromium have been reported to cause kidney problems.

Amino acids are the basic structure units of proteins. Some researchers have a theory that increasing the available amino acids decreases the loss of proteins in muscle during exercise. Again, for the golfer there is no evidence that extra amino acids enhance your strength or increase the length of your drives.

Dehydroepiandrosterone (DHEA) is found in wild yams. This chemical is a precursor to steroids. The thought is that DHEA will increase the production of testosterone and provide an anabolic steroid effect. This drug may increase the risk of uterine or prostate cancer. There is no evidence that DHEA enhances athletic performance, and its safety needs to be questioned.

Who should take supplements? First, there is no evidence that vitamin supplements enhance athletic performance, increase strength, build muscles, or improve endurance. Outright vitamin deficiency is rare. Vitamin supplements may be appropriate for certain dieters who restrict food intake to less than 1200 calories per day. Individuals who are lactose intolerant or unable to digest milk may benefit from a calcium supplement. Some individuals have food allergies and would benefit from a vitamin supplement. Vegetarians who are active and eat no animal foods may be deficient in vitamin B12 and riboflavin.

If you have been persuaded by marketing campaigns and are taking vitamins, choose a multiple vitamin with 100 percent of daily values. A multiple vitamin is preferable to large doses of single vitamins. Also, keep in mind that store brands are likely to be identical to name brands and are much less expensive.

Energy Bars

Energy bars are a popular source of carbohydrates. These supplements are high in calories, from 150 to 230 per bar. If you frequently feel hungry when you play golf, consider snacking throughout your round on dried fruits, pretzels, or low-fat granola bars—instead of the high-calorie bars.

In our foursome, there is always at least one golfer who has had a difficult front nine and is desperately looking for a quick fix at the turn to boost his or her energy level. In a matter of seconds, the glove is off and the nearest candy bar or cookie is devoured. Unfortunately, these high-sugar foods may impair performance. Following a large dose of sugar, the body triggers an insulin response to lower the sugar, resulting in fatigue and loss of concentration. The medical term is hypoglycemia. If you need a quick fix, substitute fruit (bananas or oranges), which will not trigger this insulin response.

Energy-based bars contain fructose and not the sugar glucose (found in candy), so the insulin response is not triggered.

myth & TRUTHS

Myth: A candy bar or a sugar drink helps golfers regain focus.

Truth: A high sugar load may temporarily make you feel better, but later in the round you may have a rebound effect with a dramatic drop in your sugar and a major loss of focus. Look to fruit or frequent snacking to prevent hypoglycemia and the possible rebound effect that comes with a high sugar load.

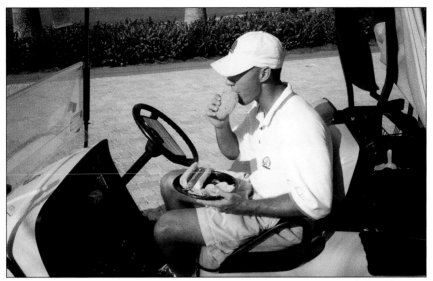

An unhealthy snack at the turn

Caffeine

Many of us have a cup or two of coffee before we begin our round and often grab a soda at the turn. Caffeine is a mild stimulant that lasts only a few hours. Caffeine affects each individual's performance differently. Some golfers thrive on it, while others are unable to putt because of jitters. One should avoid excess coffee prior to playing (no more than two cups). Not only may it cause tremors, but caffeine also has a diuretic effect—it increases urine formation. For this reason, coffee and soda should not be used for fluid replacement, stick to water.

If you want to optimize your performance, think diet and nutrition. Eat the right foods and avoid dehydration. This will result in more energy and less fatigue, enabling you to focus and excel on those finishing holes. PGA Tour players have become more conscious of proper conditioning, exercise, and nutrition. Payne Stewart is one professional who has enlisted a personal nutritionist to help him with his diet.

As the NCAA guidelines state, "there are no shortcuts to sound nutrition and the use of suspected or advertised supplemental aids may be detrimental and in most cases provide no competitive advantage."

Health Tip: Snacking on low-fat foods throughout the round may be better than eating a quick-fix energy bar.
• Yogurt contains all the nutrients of whole milk but less fat and cholesterol.
• Bananas are high in carbohydrates to fuel muscles.
• Whole-grain breads and bagels are excellent sources of carbohydrates.

Links to Experience

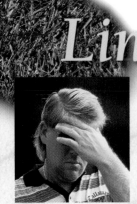

John Daly

The career of talented John Daly has been in shambles because of alcohol-related problems. Despite rehabilitation and hospitalization at the Betty Ford Clinic, he continues his struggle with this addiction. At the Vancouver Open he experienced the shakes brought on by alcohol withdrawal. Later in Memphis, Tennessee, during his round he snapped a five iron in half. Daly said, "I still get the shakes whether I play good or bad. It makes golf very difficult, being an alcoholic."

His fellow players have continued to support him in his efforts to deal with his addiction. He is now back on tour making a comeback—both in golf and in his battle with alcohol.

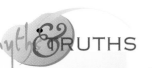

Myth: You have had a bad front nine because you felt "tight" so a beer at the turn will help.

Truth: Alcohol will not only decrease your ability to concentrate but will increase the likelihood of dehydration because of its effect on the kidneys. You may find that you are more concerned about looking for a bathroom after your beer than hitting your next shot.

The 19th Hole: Alcohol

If you have a few bad holes on the front side and you grab a "beer or two" at the turn to relax, don't expect great things to happen when you resume playing. Beer, like all alcohol, will cause you to lose focus. It also has a diuretic effect that will increase your need to urinate—and that can affect your concentration. It also impairs your visual perception and muscle coordination.

To excel in golf requires course management; extend that to the 19th hole. The 19th hole is the traditional place to analyze the round. It's a time for you and your opponents or partner to hash over the "should have been," "could have been," and "would have been" shots of the day, collect on the Nassau, and plan your next round.

The setting for this intense psychoanalytic session is generally the grill room or patio, where we often observe fellow golfers struggling over the same misfortunes. These soul-searching discussions are frequently accompanied by a beverage or two.

An occasional beer after a round is an enjoyable way to share a golf tale and celebrate a round of golf on a beautiful course. The problem arises when the occasional beer turns into four or five. Instead of having a drink to share the events of the day with friends, it is used to forget the round. Both beer and "hard liquor" have alcoholic and toxic effects. Spending too much time at the 19th hole can have a negative impact on your golf game.

If you abuse alcohol, you may run the risk of losing not only the match but also your life. Alcohol affects the liver, brain, and heart. One of the common problems on the golf course is heart palpitations after drinking alcohol. Some golfers, after several drinks, develop a rapid irregular heart rhythm. It is not easy to putt the ball, much less concentrate, if your heart rate is doubled. The phenomenon of palpitations due to excessive alcohol consumption is common during Christmas and Thanksgiving season and often termed "holiday heart." Long-term use of alcohol can affect your heart muscle by reducing its pumping capacity. This impairs your ability to maintain adequate energy on the back nine. Thirsty on the course? Grab a bottle of water instead of a beer from the beverage cart.

Alcohol can be enjoyed in moderation. Unfortunately, for some it can have disastrous effects. Tour players Brian Barnes and John Daly are examples of players who have had significant problems.

myth & TRUTHS

Myth: Sodas can be substituted for coffee since they have little caffeine.
Truth: Coffee has approximately 230 mg of caffeine and sodas contain 30 to 50 mg per can — yes, this still can give you the jitters.

If you drink, don't drive. Don't even putt.
Dean Martin

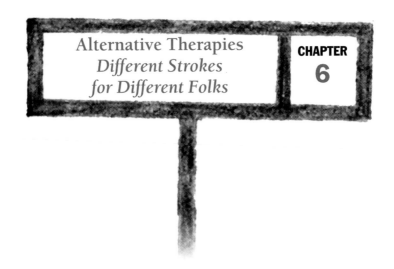

There is no question that the mind plays a major role in the body's response to medicine or intervention. The role of alternative therapies for treatment of pain remains unclear. It is important that everyone maintain an open mind and encourage scientific studies to verify their effectiveness. It is equally important to ensure that alternative therapies cause no harm.

Are Magnets for You?

Given the advertising, infomercials, and testimonials, one would think that magnets can do everything from alleviating pain and providing energy to correcting your slice and lowering your handicap.

The medical benefits of magnets have been touted by the Chinese as far back as 2000 B.C., by Hippocrates in ancient Greece and, more recently, by Jim Colbert of the Senior Tour and quarterback Dan Marino.

Magnets are claimed to have "healing power" and are available in arm and leg wraps, shoes, belts, braces, and bracelets. Theoretically these work by increasing the circulation of blood. To date, there is little scientific evidence that magnets work in this manner or have healing power. The best study to date is from the researchers at Baylor College of Medicine in Texas.[2] A magnetic device was found to reduce pain in seventy-six percent of post-polio patients, as compared to nineteen percent in patients treated with a placebo. Neither group knew who had magnet therapy and who had fake (placebo) magnets. Although the study suggested a positive benefit, it should be considered preliminary and not conclusive.

Full endorsement of this therapy will need to await further studies that are now being funded by the National Institute of Health.

For those who believe in magnet therapy, the good news is that there is no evidence to show that they do not work, nor is there any evidence to suggest that they are harmful.

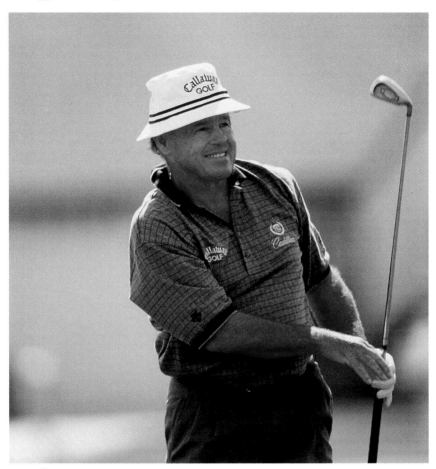

Jim Colbert

Copper Bracelets

Advocates of copper bracelets, and now copper watches, are touting the bracelets as a remedy for arthritis pain. The bracelets, which are worn on the wrist, reportedly work when the copper dissolves and enters the body by absorption through the skin. The hypothesis is that many golfers do not take in enough copper in their diet and that supplemental copper can ease the pain from arthritis.

To date there is no scientific evidence that supports these claims; however, as with magnets, there is also no evidence that they cause any harm.

Antioxidants — the Super Vitamins

Antioxidants are known to have many important health benefits, but can they improve your golf game? The answer may be yes. The antioxidant vitamins C and E protect the cells of the body from damage by "free radicals." Some of these super antioxidants have been shown to improve blood circulation and enhance exercise endurance. In one scientific study, pycnogenol, an antioxidant derived from the bark of a French pine tree, increased endurance in both male and female recreational athletes.[3] There is no evidence that it can improve strength or focus, but it may prevent damage to the muscle cells of your arms and legs.

Herbal Remedies

You have most likely seen or heard the advertisements proclaiming herbal remedies as the natural way to health. Health food companies sell energy bars with herbs and vitamins to golfers by professing increased concentration, energy, and improved calmness. But do they work? While we may be depressed about our golf game, it remains unclear whether St. John's Wort, the "natural Prozac," will make us feel any better about our double bogies on the last three holes. And will Ginkgo Biloba, the dementia-fighting herb and memory enhancer, assist your opponent in recalling that he or she had a six and not a five on that last hole? Researchers need to do more work before we'll know for sure.

Some other popular herbs include:

- Bilbery for eye health
- Boswellia as an anti-inflammatory
- Horse chestnut for circulation
- Kava for anxiety and maybe the yips
- Aloe vera for burns, wound healing, and skin irritations
- Echinacea for reduction of common cold symptoms and immune stimulus
- Garlic for its antibacterial and antifungal properties

If you elect to take herbs, remember that because it is natural does not mean it is safe. Herbs and prescription medications can have interactions that may be harmful. Because there is little regulation and standardization of "herbal therapies," the herb content and efficacy of different preparations may vary among different manufacturers.

If you do use herbal therapies, more is not better. Stick with the recommended dosages. Since there is a lack of studies regarding long-term use, these supplements should be used for only a few weeks at a time.

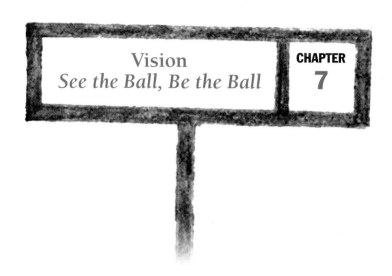

Vision
See the Ball, Be the Ball

CHAPTER 7

Most people play a fair game of golf — if you watch them.

— Joey Adams

In our valiant attempt to seek the Holy Grail in golf—a lower handicap—we leave no stone unturned. Big-headed clubs, space-age shafts, and magnets for our bodies are used in desperation to improve our game.

And yet, if you are one of the millions of golfers who wear prescription glasses, you may be overlooking an essential piece of equipment that is a major factor in your game—your glasses. In fact, they may be a handicap.

Corrective Eyewear

After going through my third putter in as many years, my Pro suggested that maybe the problem was with my sight and not my stroke. At age fifty, like millions of golfers, I wear prescription glasses. After discussing this explanation about poor putting with my colleagues who deal with visual problems, I learned that the golfer, especially the golfer with bifocals, may have problems with image displacement (the ball is not really where you think it is). Depending on our head position, we may be looking through the lens in an off-center part, causing displacement or, as ophthalmologists and optometrists refer to it, the prismatic effect. It depends on your lens prescription. If you are nearsighted, the ball will be farther from the feet; if you are farsighted, the ball will be closer to the feet. You could be swinging at something that is not really there.

43

For many of us, wearing eyeglasses may be a handicap to our game. My playing partner kept taking his glasses off when he putted. Always looking for a good tip, I asked him if he could see better without them. He remarked he could see better with them, but when looking toward the hole, the edge of the frame would get in the way. Sam Snead once commented, after a round of golf with Eisenhower, that the President could play better if he got bigger glasses. "I think the edge of his frame gets in the way of his vision on his backswing." On today's tour, players prefer large frames to increase their field of vision. Because putting involves good peripheral vision, glasses should be large with a thin rim and a face/form shape. Temples should not be wide or on line. Depth perception and the ability to determine texture when reading greens are important in golf.

Health Tip
Contact lenses may increase glare. It's highly recommended that you wear sunglasses.

Bifocals may result in visual distortion. Some golfers may find benefits in wearing a single-vision lens or mini-bifocals. If the second lens is placed at the lower right-hand corner, it will keep the segment (line) out of the way on the backswing. Adapting the lens to the sport uses the advantage of bifocals. The wearer can see the ball land on the green *and* read the scorecard.

Contact Lenses

Another option to help you see your shot more clearly is the use of contact lenses. Golf is played in all weather conditions—wind, rain, heat, and cold. Contacts not only allow us to see better in these conditions, but enable us to avoid perspiration dripping on our glasses in hot weather. Many serious golfers wear soft contact lenses that are inserted daily. The environment in which we play exposes us to wind and dust. Playing in areas of the country with low humidity or wind will result in drying of the lenses, leading to irritation of the eyes. Frequent lubrication with saline drops will help the lenses keep their shape and keep the ball in focus. Small saline bottles in your bag may be just as important as balls, tees, and gloves. The larger soft lenses with larger optic zones are less likely to dislocate.

Golfers who wear contact lenses can opt for monovision. This technique uses the dominant eye set for distance and the nondominant eye set for a closer distance, that is, from the eyes to the ground for putting. Monovision may work well if you play the same course, but different courses will require improved depth perception. This may require an adjustment with a third lens.

Laser Surgery

With recent advances in technology, the cornea can now be reshaped with the use of a laser. This new technique may enable you to play golf without glasses, as in the case of PGA and LPGA professionals like Fred Funk, Tom Kite, and Kris Tschetter.

Since the cornea is responsible for approximately seventy percent of the eye's ability to bend and focus light, most procedures attempt to alter the way your eye focuses light by changing the shape of your cornea.

The Excimer laser works by emitting ultraviolet light and high-energy pulses that last only a billionth of a second to disrupt the molecular bonds of the cornea and thus change its shape. The laser beam is not hot and does not cause damage to surrounding tissues. Stitches are not usually required.

The surgery is designed to eliminate the need for glasses but does not always create 20/20 or 20/40 vision.

Laser surgery is not for everyone and it is generally performed on one eye at a time. If glasses and contacts continue to interfere with your game, consult your ophthalmologist and see if this procedure can help your score.

Sunglasses

If you play frequently and live in areas of the country where the sun is strong, you may need to take extra precaution by wearing sunglasses. Eyes, like our skin, can be affected by ultraviolet light radiation emitted by sunlight. Cataract formation and damage to the retina may result from

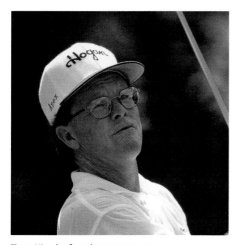

Tom Kite before laser surgery

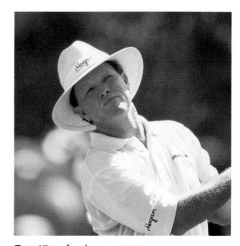

Tom Kite after laser surgery

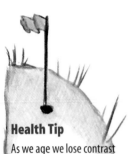

UV rays and lead to blindness. Glare causes us to squint, tensing our facial muscles at a time when we are trying to get our body to relax. Pterygium—growths on the white part of the eye—occur from overexposure to sunlight. It feels like a piece of dirt or gravel in the eye. This may require surgical removal, as in the case of PGA professional Gary Koch. Sunglasses can block out the harmful effects of the sun's rays. Annika Sorenstam and David Duval are part of a growing group of professionals who choose to protect their eyes from the harmful effects of the sun, wind, and sand.

What to Look for in Sunglasses

Some eighty to ninety percent of the harmful UVB light can be eliminated, depending on the quality and shape of the lens. In choosing sunglasses, you want a pair that reduces glare and ultraviolet light and at the same time does not distort colors, which can affect one's ability to read greens.

In order not to affect depth perception, especially in reading breaks on the green, choose sunglasses that have an ellipsoid or wraparound lens. These will minimize distortion of your peripheral vision.

Choose a pair that changes color minimally. We need to select the right color lenses for the conditions in which we are playing. Gray lenses have the least effect on distortion of normal colors and are the best choice to preserve natural contrast. Brown and orange lenses provide better contrast for seeing the ball against the sky but are likely to distort the color green needed to read those subtle changes in the green. The brown-shaded lenses also make it easier for players like me to find that white ball in the heavy green rough. Because conditions vary you might consider the use of interchangeable lenses. If it's sunny, wear cinnamon-colored lenses and if cloudy, choose lenses that are yellow or rose.

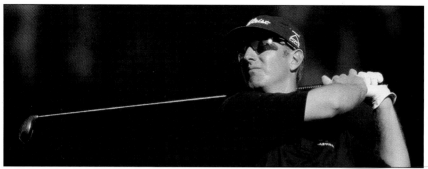

David Duval

Which Tints?
Tinted lenses have what are called absorption and transmission qualities. What the tint does not absorb, the eye receives. Filtered by lenses, the light the eye receives helps golfers discriminate between subtle slopes and contours to varying degrees. Below are descriptions of common tints from Bollé, with individual attributes.

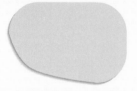

Yellow absorbs 14 percent of visible light transmission (VLT), and is preferred for cloudy days.

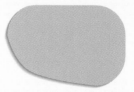

Vermillion absorbs 50 percent of VLT, and is preferred for use on cloudy days.

Cinnamon absorbs 54 percent of VLT, and is the most popular tint among players tested.

Citrus absorbs 65 percent of VLT. It is popular on sunnier days, and is also rated highly by players tested.

Gray absorbs 74 of VLT. This tint was least liked by players tested.

VISUAL PROBLEMS: WHAT YOU SHOULD KNOW

- Harmful effects of the sun may cause cataracts or damage the retina.
- Glasses, especially bifocals, may distort the position of the ball.
- Hats and visors may reduce glare, but are minimally effective in reducing UV light, resulting in an SPF of two.

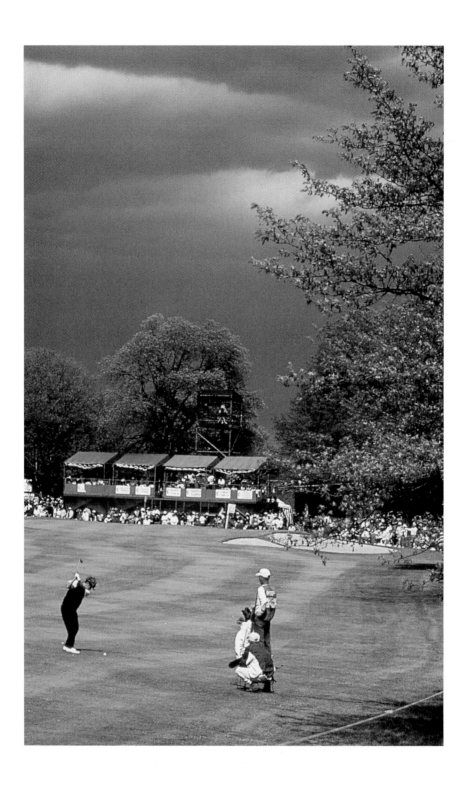

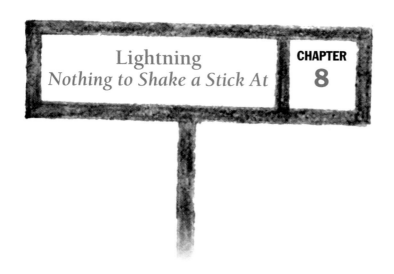

| Lightning
Nothing to Shake a Stick At | CHAPTER
8 |

When God wants to play through, you let Him play through.

—Lee Trevino

Lightning isn't on the average person's list of things to worry about. Most people see lightning as a sky spectacle, viewed from the safety of their homes or cars. They know it's dangerous, but it's a danger on a par with cyclones, tornadoes, and flash floods—it'll never happen to them.

Golfers know differently. Standing in an open field holding a metal club is as vulnerable as one can be during a lightning storm—precisely the position many golfers have found themselves in.

Both the USGA and the PGA take lightning seriously enough to have gone to the considerable trouble and expense of installing storm monitoring systems at all of the major tournament sites. Current equipment can detect lightning up to two hundred miles away. Lightning detection instruments, the size of a cellular phone, are now available for the individual golfer and can detect lightning up to forty miles away.

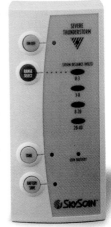

A hand-held lightning detector

As forces of nature go, lightning is a serious adversary. A form of high-voltage electric discharge, its temperature can reach up to 60,000°F. Hit directly by a lightning bolt, one in three people will die. If you are not killed, you will likely have long-term problems affecting your heart. Ruptured eardrums are common and cataracts may also develop—sometimes months or even years after the fact. You might also sustain neuropsychiatric injuries that develop slowly.

51

The jolt of electricity the victim of a lightning strike sustains can disrupt the respiratory system, causing breathing to slow or even stop. The heart frequently develops an irregular rhythm, occasionally escalating into a wildly disordered pattern known as ventricular fibrillation, which may lead to cardiac arrest and death. In addition to skin burns, muscle damage, fractures, and internal injuries can occur as a result of the person's being thrown to the ground by the force of the strike.

myth&RUTHS

Myth: Although lightning is off in the distance, I am protected while sitting in a golf cart because it has rubber tires. My umbrella has a fiberglass shaft and, therefore, I am unlikely to get struck.
Truth: An open golf cart provides no protection, although a shielded automobile would. If your fiberglass umbrella is the tallest object in the area, it may be the site of the strike.

Victims of lightning strikes typically lose consciousness, become confused, and often have periods of amnesia. It is not uncommon to have total amnesia regarding the events surrounding the lightning strike. Because of this confusion, a person who has been struck by lightning may regain consciousness and insist that he or she is fine. In point of fact, he or she needs immediate medical attention. Remember that there is no truth to the myth that the victim remains charged after being struck by lightning.

Golfers face a greater than average risk of being struck by lightning. A look at the statistics shows that people who got hit tended to be out in an open field on a late Sunday afternoon in July. Sound familiar? With all of its golf courses, Florida has twice as many lightning deaths and injuries as any other state. A single storm front moving across the state can produce 20,000 strikes. Storms can come up suddenly and without warning, and the nature of the sport demands that its participants will often be at some distance from any adequate shelter. And, of course, the metal rods they carry turn innocent golfers into virtual lightning rods.

Over the years there have been many harrowing tales of lightning strikes on the golf course. In 1975, at the U.S. Open in Chicago, three men—Lee Trevino, Bobby Nichols, and Jerry Head—were struck simultaneously. Trevino actually had four burn spots on his shoulder where the bolt left his body. Presumably, he didn't follow his own tongue-in-cheek advice to hold up a 1-iron in a storm "because even God couldn't hit a 1-iron."

At the U.S. Open at Hazeltine, it was the spectators who were hit—this time by a "splash" strike (a splash is a kind of spillover strike: the primary site is elsewhere while the splash hits those nearby). A splash strike is not a gentle little "leftover," however! In another case, one golfer was struck while standing on the green holding a flag stick. His partner got the splash; it knocked him right off his feet and hurled him a distance of nearly ten feet.

Finding a safe spot can be a problem on the golf course. During the PGA championships at Shoal Creek, a storm set in that was strong enough for officials to issue a warning. The tournament's administrator took shelter in one of the trailers. He picked up the phone to make a call, and suddenly found himself slammed against the trailer door. His breathing was labored and shallow, and he had no feeling in his arms or legs. Lightning had struck both the trailer and the telephone transformer, literally leaving him with no place to hide and no way to call for help. Luckily, EMTs were on the scene immediately and he was rushed to the hospital where he made a full recovery.

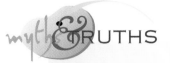

Myth: When out on the golf course and lightning is approaching, remove golf shoes because they have metal spikes.

Truth: There is little likelihood that spiked golfing shoes will increase the chance of getting struck. Keep shoes on and get off the course quickly.

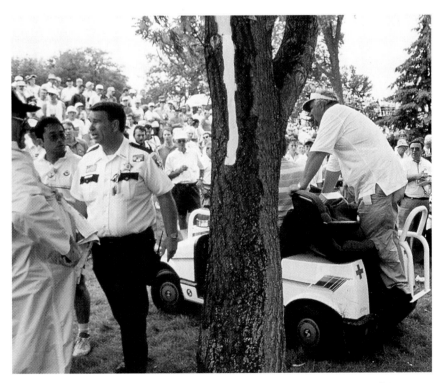

The 1991 U.S. Open at Hazeltine—emergency personnel work at the scene of the lightning strike.

Incidents like these have led tournament officials to err on the side of caution. If lightning is within twenty-five miles and approaching, play may be suspended. In such a case, Rule 6-8B requires players to stop immediately only if they are "between the play of two holes." The rule allows those in the process of playing a hole to continue, provided they do so without delay.

If you do continue to play, it is not necessary that you finish the hole if conditions worsen. However, once you stop, you must stop for good. You cannot change your mind and finish the hole. The penalty for a breech of Rule 6-8B in match or stroke play is disqualification. Rule 6-8C allows you to mark and lift your ball in order that it not be washed or blown away. Rule 6-8A allows a golfer to discontinue play on his or her own if he or she believes there is danger from lightning. Play must, however, be resumed when ordered by the committee.

Links to Experience

Melvin Febres, a fourteen-year-old-boy, was performing maintenance on the golf course with his cousin when threatening weather appeared. They sought shelter under an isolated tree. Lightning struck the tree and the splash strike hit both boys. Melvin was unconscious and his cousin was knocked to the ground and lost hearing in one ear. Dennis Rockwell, a member of golf Security, was the first one to arrive on the scene. He said, "When I got there, he (Melvin) wasn't breathing and he didn't have a pulse." Using an automatic external defibrillator, or AED, he shocked Melvin back to life and then started CPR. Melvin was then taken by ambulance to the hospital for further treatment and observation. (See Chapter 12 for more information about AEDs.)

LIGHTNING: WHAT YOU SHOULD KNOW

When dealing with lightning, as in medicine, prevention is better than cure. Following a few simple guidelines will substantially reduce your risk of receiving a bolt from the blue.

■ Thunderstorms develop quickly. If you hear thunder, don't waste time calculating the distance the lightning must travel to get to you or the likelihood of your being struck; you are already within range of the next flash. Get off the course. Many courses sound an alarm to warn golfers of approaching storms. Heed the warnings; get off the course.

■ Avoid isolated trees. Lone trees may attract lightning rather than protect you from it. You are better off seeking shelter in a dense wooded area.

■ If caught in open fairway, and lightning is imminent, drop to your knees but minimize contact with the ground. Maintain balance and do not touch the ground with your hands; electricity can be conducted over wet fairways.

■ Get rid of umbrellas, both metal and fiberglass, as well as clubs and the flag stick. These must now be considered lightning rods.

■ Water serves as an excellent conductor of electricity; avoid ponds and puddles.

■ Do not be the highest object on the horizon. Choose low-lying areas over hilltops (bunkers are a good bet).

■ The golf cart has rubber tires but minimal shielding and should not be considered a safe area. An automobile is a much wiser choice.

■ If lightning is near, the hair on your neck and arms may "stand on end." This is evidence of increased electrical difference between your body and the cloud. You should run from the area as quickly as possible and then drop to your knees without touching the ground with your hands.

■ If an individual has been struck by lightning and is unresponsive, the first person on the scene, referred to as the initial responder, should begin CPR (see Appendix) and send someone to the clubhouse for the automatic external defibrillator, or AED, if the course has one. (See Chapter 12.)

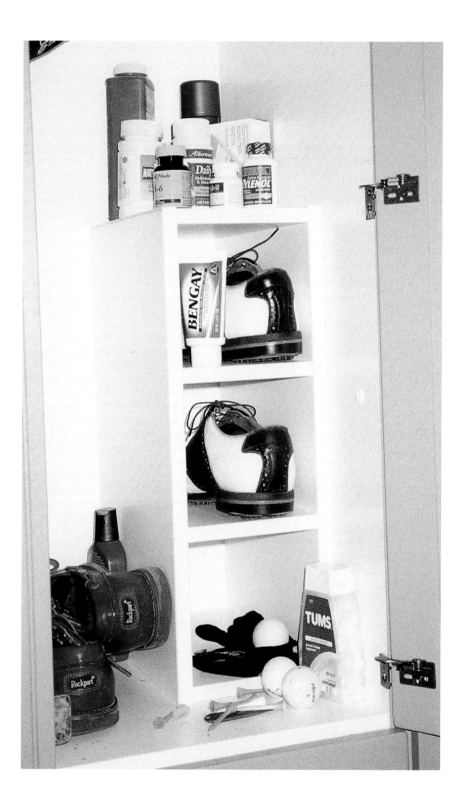

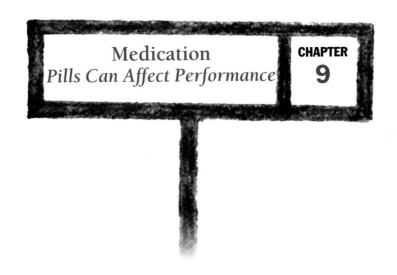

| Medication | CHAPTER |
| Pills Can Affect Performance | 9 |

Every cure is temporary, but it's nice while it lasts.

—Jack Nicklaus

Once you get hooked on golf, you soon realize that the rest of your life has to be readjusted. Four to five hours on the course, plus the time it takes to get there and back (not to mention the time spent in the club afterwards!), means a big chunk of your day. Mealtimes may need to be rearranged, and even sleeping habits may have to change. And if you, like millions of other Americans, take medications daily, you may find that your old dosage schedule doesn't suit you on the days you play golf.

You select your clubs meticulously, considering factors like weight, grip, and length to determine which one is right for a particular shot. Your body deserves at least the same consideration; keeping in mind the fact that you will be on your feet for at least four hours, when is the best time to take your medicines? Will a particular drug affect your concentration? If you have a beer as a chaser, will the mixture cause problems while you are driving back home?

High Blood Pressure Medications

Let's start with high blood pressure medication, since most golfers, at one time or another, claim that the sport sends theirs sky high. One of the most common drugs used to keep high blood pressure under control is the diuretic, which acts on the kidneys to increase the production of urine, thus reducing the volume of blood in the body. This is important to lessen the strain on the heart, which is actually the organ we are most concerned with when treating high blood pressure. For our purposes here, however, the main thing to know about diuretics is that you will have to urinate more frequently when you are taking them. This presents the obvious practical problem of needing to be near a bathroom, as well as the question of dehydration in hot weather. (Heat illness is discussed fully in Chapter 4.) The simplest measure may be to take your medication after rather than before you start your round, thus avoiding the whole issue.

Beta-Blockers

Another type of high blood pressure medication is the group known as beta-blockers (Inderal, Lopressor, Atenolol), which are also prescribed for people with coronary heart disease. These agents slow the heart rate and block the action of adrenaline, the hormone our bodies produce in times of stress and exertion. This reduces of the heart's need for oxygen, making it easier for people with hypertension or heart disease to carry on a normal existence.

One of the beneficial side effects of the beta-blockers is that they reduce anxiety and tremors. Classical musicians have been known to use them before a major performance, and a recent study confirms that students who took this drug before taking their SAT exams scored higher marks as a result. Indeed, taking beta-blockers improves steadiness to such an extent that they have been banned in such sports as archery and shooting. In golf, beta-blockers have been used by such players as Larry Laoretti, Nick Price, and Mac O'Grady, all with equivocal results. There is no evidence that they are in widespread use on tour, nor are they banned by the USGA.

. . . for many heart patients, the exercise, fresh air, and the pleasure of playing are 'just what the doctor ordered.'

In the United Kingdom, however, the government body Sports Council encourages drug testing for golfers and specifically forbids the use of performance-enhancing drugs while competing in the British Open. Its list of drugs does include beta-blockers.

While we are on the subject of the heart, let me repeat what I have said in other chapters: heart problems are no reason to give up the game. Many people who have had heart attacks, bypass surgery, or pacemakers implanted still play frequently and with single-digit handicaps. Indeed, for many heart patients, the exercise, fresh air, and the pleasure of playing are "just what the doctor ordered."

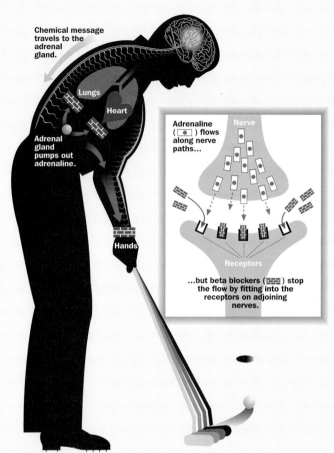

Chemical message travels to the adrenal gland.

Lungs

Heart

Adrenal gland pumps out adrenaline.

Hands

Adrenaline (⬚) flows along nerve paths...

Nerve

Receptors

...but beta blockers (▦) stop the flow by fitting into the receptors on adjoining nerves.

How beta-blockers work

When you get nervous or frightened, the brain responds by sending "fight-or-flight" messages down the spinal cord and sympathetic nervous system to the rest of the body. These chemical messages are mediated by the secretion of adrenaline. Also known as epinephrine, adrenaline is the main hormone that causes such physiological alarms as the heart to beat faster, the palms to sweat, and the hands to tremble. Adrenaline triggers these changes in the individual cells via entry points known as beta-receptors. Because their chemical structure is very similar to that of adrenaline, beta-blocking drugs are able to attach to the receptors instead, thereby preventing the adrenaline from delivering its anxiety-provoking message.

If you are taking cardiac medication, however, be sure you are following your doctor's orders here as well! Some medications, especially the ones that control the heart's rhythm, must be taken exactly as directed. In other words, don't wait until the end of the round, or try to juggle your pill with your stint in the club. These drugs are effective only for a limited period, after which you are, essentially, on your own. Golf has its own sense of time and, without a conscious effort, you may find that your pill-popping hour has come and gone while you were busy gazing meditatively across the fairway or cursing your luck for landing in a bunker. Come up with a system that ensures you remember to take your medicine at the proper time.

Health Tip: If you're on any medication, ask your physician before taking vitamins and mineral supplements; they can interact with other drugs.

Nonsteroidal Anti-Inflammatories (NSAIDs)

Since we all don't possess the picture-perfect turn of Tiger Woods and our swing mechanics can be described best as "not quite fluid," we often suffer injury and pain.

Most golfers choose anti-inflammatories for pain relief. Today billions of dollars are spent for prescription and over the counter nonsteroidal anti-inflamatories (NSAIDs). These medications, which include ibuprofen, naproxen, and aspirin, can reduce inflammation and provide analgesia. Ibuprofen that you purchase without a prescription is a dose of 200 mg; by prescription, strengths of 400 mg and 800 mg are available. The average dose for pain relief is 400 mg every four to six hours. Dosages higher than 400 mg are not likely to provide more pain relief and can be harmful. Side effects can and do occur, especially if you have kidney or liver disease.

> *Many amateurs have a tendency to overdo instruction. It's like the old saying, 'A couple of aspirin might cure you, but the whole bottle will probably kill you.'*
>
> Sam Snead

Ritalin

The medication Ritalin is known to enhance a person's ability to focus. This stimulant is used for the treatment of Attention Deficit Disorder (ADD). Initially thought to be found just in children, ADD is now well recognized in the adult population. Payne Stewart was diagnosed with ADD because of his easy distractibility and loss of focus. After diagnostic testing, he was placed on Ritalin to facilitate the proper interaction of his brain chemistries (brain neurotransmitter substances). Although a trial of Ritalin did not improve his ability to concentrate, it is helpful for many people with this disorder.

Ritalin is a carefully controlled prescription drug and indicated for those with a proven diagnosis of ADD. There is no evidence that this medication will enhance concentration or focus in individuals without ADD who have normal brain chemistries. Stewart won the 1999 U.S. Open in a dramatic eighteenth-hole finish, despite not having taken Ritalin. A characteristic of individuals who have ADD is not only easy distractibility, but the capacity to focus excessively. Payne was able to take his minor disability and turn it into an advantage, demonstrating intense concentration during the final round.

Health Tip: If you are dehydrated, you should replace your fluids before taking NSAIDs because of possible side effects.

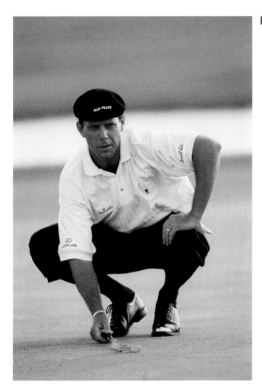
Payne Stewart

Nitroglycerin

Nitroglycerin, or NTG, is a vasodilator, a drug that makes the blood vessels wider, and the speed with which it works to relieve the pain of angina is nothing short of amazing. Many heart patients make it a habit to carry nitroglycerin tablets wherever they go and to use them in advance of situations where they anticipate experiencing chest discomfort. If activities like climbing hills or walking in hot weather cause you chest pain or tightness, and your physician has prescribed nitroglycerin, you may want to try taking it before the discomfort occurs. Check with your physician before trying this, however. In addition, since anxiety and stress can also induce angina, consider taking nitroglycerin if you intend to compete in a tournament, or before a particularly crucial shot. Again, check with your physician. You can make nitroglycerin a standard item in your golf bag, along with your sunscreen and your water bottle. Be sure, however, that your prescription is kept up to date—the speed with which these tablets lose their potency seems in direct proportion to the speed with which they relieve pain. They can become useless in a matter of two or three months, particularly if they are not stored in a cool place.

Nitroglycerin is taken by placing it under the tongue, where it dissolves and is absorbed into the circulation. After you take your NTG, you should stop and rest for five to ten minutes, until the discomfort has gone, before resuming your golf. If you have angina and have been prescribed NTG, consider telling your playing partners how they can help you take your NTG if you need assistance. Let them know that if there is no relief after two or three NTG doses, they should send someone in the group back to the pro shop to call 911 or your local emergency number.

Drugs and Photosensitivity

Of particular interest to golfers is the tendency of certain medications (and some perfumes and cosmetics as well) to cause a skin reaction when exposed to the sun. This is known as photosensitivity and the reaction, which appears as a fierce red sunburn, is generally limited to the skin that is actually exposed. Unfortunately, susceptibility to photosensitivity increases with age.

Medications with this side effect span a wide range of commonly prescribed drugs including some for diabetes, hypertension, and heart disease. Antibiotics, such as the sulfas and tetracycline, can also cause a reaction, as can nonsteroidal anti-inflammatories (used to treat minor arthritis and muscle aches) like Naprosyn, Feldene, and Clinoril. Check the label for possible side effects.

Myth: Hormone therapy can increase strength and keep our bodies from aging.
Truth: Hormone intervention is justifiable only with estrogen for the postmenopausal woman.

If you do get a photosensitive reaction, treat it as you would an ordinary sunburn. Cold water compresses and cool baths will ease your discomfort, and avoiding the sun as much as possible will prevent it from worsening. The suggestions in Chapter 3 on preventing skin cancer certainly apply here as well. The main point is to protect your skin in every way possible, including the conscientious use of sunscreen, long sleeves and pants, and wide-brimmed hats. It also helps to avoid being outdoors during peak sun time.

Keep in mind that virtually every drug has side effects. If photosensitivity becomes too difficult to bear, discuss the possibility of an alternative medication with your physician.

Steroids

The desire for greater athletic achievement has resulted in a dramatic increase in drug usage. Anabolic steroids are used primarily by power athletes (weight lifters, football players) and endurance athletes (swimmers, distance runners). These dangerous drugs have not been seen on the golf tour. Anabolic steroids enhance certain physiologic functions including lean body mass, strength, and a reduction in recovery time between workouts. They also enhance irritability and aggressiveness. The side effects of using these steroids include hepatitis, leukemia, and even the development of tumors. Since steroids increase your body mass and make you prone to outbursts of anger, it makes sense that this combination makes them unsuitable for the golfer.

MEDICATIONS: WHAT YOU SHOULD KNOW

- Beta-blockers are used for cardiac patients and as a treatment for high blood pressure. They are known to improve steadiness and reduce tremors.
- Nitroglycerin is a tablet placed under the tongue to relieve chest discomfort associated with heart problems.
- Anabolic steroids increase strength and aggressiveness and are not helpful for the golfer.
- Certain antibiotics and diuretics may cause a photosensitive (sunburn type) reaction if the individual is exposed to the sun.
- Ritalin may enhance focus and concentration but only in those individuals diagnosed with Attention Deficit Disorder (ADD).
- Never take medication with alcohol.
- Nonsteroidal anti-inflammatories (NSAIDs), such as ibuprofen, should be taken with food because they can irritate the stomach lining.

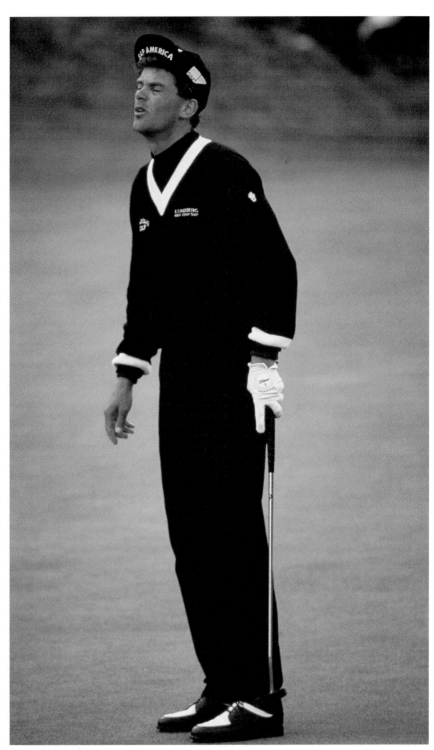

Jesper Parnevik

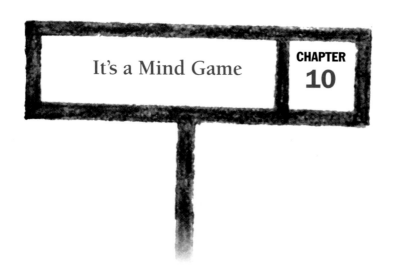

It's a Mind Game

The mind messes up more shots than the body.

—Tommy Bolt

What is it about hitting a stationary white ball that engenders such emotional responses of fear, frustration, anxiety, anger, and incredible joy? Golf is different from most sports. It is long in duration, requiring mental concentration for some four to five hours. You play the ball less than one percent of the time. By comparison, in tennis you play the ball more than twenty-five percent of the time. Golf allows long periods of time in which it is easy to lose concentration and become distracted. In a match, we are not allowed a coach or time-out to regroup. Substitutes cannot provide relief if we are in a slump for a few holes. If our opponent is in the zone, hitting shots from all over the course, we cannot play defensively, as in other sports, by blocking shots. In golf, we are alone with our emotions. Our ability to deal with and manage our emotions determines our success.

Dr. Tim Gallwey, author of *The Inner Game of Golf*, feels that players are "saddled with self-doubt, lapses in concentration, self-anger and low self-esteem, which are more likely to prevent them from reaching their scoring potential than any swing flaws."

Concentration

The game of golf requires us to concentrate and focus for eighteen holes. The golfer needs to be attentive to each and every shot. Business matters should be left at the office. Your cellular phone may be disruptive to your game and certainly a distraction to your partners.

The level and style of concentration differ among individuals. Golfers like Fuzzy Zoeller and Lee Trevino talk, joke, and interact with the gallery as they make their way through the round. They have the capacity, however, to become acutely focused when it is time to strike the ball. This type of golfer has a "trigger" or preshot routine that enables him or her to regain focus.

Curtis Strange maintains unbroken concentration during his entire round. Ben Hogan, as well, had a reputation for being able to block out anything that did not pertain to his game. A story goes that during a match his partner aced a par three. Upon reaching the next tee, Hogan asked him what he got on the last hole. Immersed in his own game, Hogan was oblivious to how his partner had played the hole.

> *Concentration is a fine antidote for anxiety.*
>
> Jack Nicklaus

Our concentration can be disrupted by negative self-talk. "Don't hit it in the water," or "keep it out of the woods." Remarking, "I could be a great putter if it weren't for my nerves," will not help you stroke the ball into the cup. Adversarial situations such as bad weather, lightning-fast greens, and out-and-out bad luck (as when your ball ends up in a divot), need to be regarded as challenges, not negatives.

Threats to our concentration include pressure, anxiety, and lack of confidence. We need to adopt a positive attitude. Although heavily bunkered, believe the green is there to catch your ball. Your focus needs to be on the present. Forget past shots and future holes. Poor golf relates to poor concentration. You need to be able to avoid distraction.

Confidence

Golf is a game of mistakes and frustration. Knowing how to deal with these situations improves scoring. We build confidence when we meet our level of expectation. Be realistic when you play. Don't expect to carry 220 yards of water and reach the par five behemoth in two. If you don't play golf often, you can't expect to score well. Hitting from the gold tees can make for a long day. Setting your sights unrealistically high will result in failure and disappointment when your goal is not achieved. Learn to deal with and expect poor luck, bad bounces, and missed shots. Self-criticism and yelling at yourself in anger will not foster confidence. Through practice, we can reinforce and build our confidence. The range is a place for honing both physical and mental skills.

myth & TRUTHS

Myth: Golf is a game of perfection.
Truth: Golf is really a game of errors. To win you need the lowest score despite making mistakes.

Practice with a purpose—make each shot count. Follow a plan. Use your entire preshot routine: mind set, attitude, and target. Be calm and determined during your practice sessions. Don't just beat balls at the range. Approach every shot with that same positive mental feeling you have when you hit a good ball! Finish your practice session after you have executed your shots successfully—leave with a positive feeling. As on the course, manage your practice time and don't forget your short game.

> *Faith is in your heart. Confidence is in your mind and heart. In golf true confidence will always beat blind faith.*
>
> *Harvey Penick*

Visualization

Mental imagery through the technique of visualization can improve performance and mind set. The ability to visualize the flight of the ball rolling to the green prepares one's mind with positive thoughts. Zig Ziglar, in his book *See You at the Top*, describes a great example of visualization. As a prisoner of war in Vietnam, he was placed in solitary confinement. Daily he visualized playing a round of golf at his home course. So detailed was his imagery that he even visualized his steps between shots. Upon his release, he returned home. In his first round of golf he shot seventy-four. He rarely broke ninety on the course before his incarceration. Similarly, Jack Nicklaus attributes fifty percent of his performance to the visualization process. Athletes in all sports use this technique to improve their skills.

Links to Experience

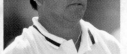

Esteban Toledo

Practicing with a passion exemplifies PGA professional Esteban Toledo, known as the Grinder King. This young Mexican continued to believe in himself. He was confident that, despite starting golf late and being self-taught, he could live his dream and qualify for the PGA Tour. As he told an Hispanic youth group, "You can do that, too, if you work hard and believe in yourself. And when you make it, you don't have to change. I am still the same inside. I am still always going to work hard."

Just as mental imagery helps create the proper mind set, rituals serve as triggers to tell our mind and body we are ready to play well. When we are under stress, our ritual patterns can be changed. We tend to rush— alter our preshot routine. No longer do we wiggle our club or walk behind the ball and visualize its flight down the fairway. The result of pressure and stress is generally to speed up and change our temper. Our backswings become quicker and we jab at our putts.

We can deal with pressure and maintain our temper by relaxing and slowing down. Take a deep breath, minimize tension in the muscles. As our arm muscles become tight, our backswings become shorter. Sam Snead once remarked, "If a lot of people gripped a knife and fork like they do a golf club they'd starve to death." The muscles in our body need to be at peace. Don't rush. Relax while walking to the next shot.

Visualize winning.

Gary Player

Stress

Golf is a solitary game. We are on our own. Anxiety begins on the first tee in front of our friends or the strangers the Starter pairs us with. There is the fear of embarrassment in missing a three-foot putt "that anybody can make." Anxiety affects both amateur and professional golfers. PGA player Hale Irwin remarked, "You start to choke when you drive through the front gate. On the first hole you just want to make contact with the ball."

The body reacts to stress by releasing the hormone adrenaline into the bloodstream. Adrenaline makes our heart go faster and our blood pressure rise. This fight-or-flight response enables our body to react to emergencies. Adrenaline is also released when a person becomes angry, frightened, or excited. The ability to deal with emotions enables us to balance the amount of adrenaline in our system. When there's too much of this hormone, we jump all over the ball (often in tournament play we hit our clubs further). On the other hand, if we don't have enough adrenaline, we lose enthusiasm and become distracted. Stress is part of the game of golf, as it is in life. Our capacity to manage it may help determine our success in the game.

Never smash a club over your opponent's head. You can't replace it under the 14 club rule.

H. Thompson

The mind needs to deal with anger, frustration, fear, and excitement. It needs to bring a positive attitude to each shot no matter what problem it presents. Anger will not cause us to concentrate more, only to lose focus and accelerate that adrenaline response.

Winning at golf, as in life, requires the virtues of patience, humility, and honesty. Course management, therefore, needs to be extended to the mind. Those who are able to master their emotions will emerge as champions.

The "Yips"

The dreaded two-foot putt conjures feelings of fear and anxiety. Immediately flashing through your mind prior to stroking the ball is "anyone can make that putt"—the putt fails to fall and you immediately feel that the yips are back. Those involuntary hand movements called the "yips" are referred to by many names including jerks, spasms, freezing, or cramps. Yips cause us to miss what we feel are the easiest of putts. This problem has been the downfall of many professional golfers and has even affected such greats as Sam Snead and Ben Hogan. The term *yips* must be derived from the exclamation that a golfer issues when he or she misses another easy putt.

> *Keep your sense of humor. There's enough stress in the rest of your life to let bad shots ruin a game you're supposed to enjoy.*
>
> — *Amy Alcott*

Yips generally only occur during putting, leaving the rest of the game unaffected. It is more likely to affect golfers who have played for a long time than novices. Missing that short putt "that anyone can make" leads to embarrassment and damage to one's pride. If we repeat this error, the fear of failure to execute a putt can influence our dominant thought process. It may reach the point where we constantly complain to our companions about our putting. The thought process becomes obsessive and almost takes on a life of its own.

One study suggested that twenty-eight percent of golfers suffer from the yips. Often it is first noted during a tournament when players are under the most pressure. It has been suggested that the affliction can add five extra shots per round.

Putting is the most frequent shot in golf; it accounts for forty percent of all shots, sometimes fifty percent in my case. Putting is different from most other shots in golf where, if you hit a poor shot, you always have the ability to recover and save par. There is no recovery from a bad putt.

> *Competitive golf is played mainly on a five-and-a-half inch course—the space between your ears.*
>
> — *Bobby Jones*

Many golfers attempt to correct the yips using "trick strategies." These tricks include changing the putter (to a longer, heavier one), using new grips, a cross-handed stroke, different stance or head position, and perhaps altering the degree of fixation on the ball. Some golfers have even tried hypnosis or Valium without success. The study on golfers with the yips noted that twenty percent had tried medication to control the affliction, all without success.

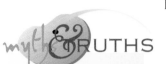

Myth: Putting Yips. The yips (a twitch, cramp, wiggle, jitter, or jerk) is a complex neurological disorder still considered incurable by the medical profession.
Truth: This phenomenon, which affects both professionals and amateurs, is not caused by nerve damage and can be overcome.

Use of large grips may be helpful. A large grip tends to reduce the activity of the wrist and finger muscles during the putting stroke. The shape can be contoured to fit in the same position every day. You should always place your hands on the grip in a consistent manner.

The yips are not the result of nerve damage or some unusual neurologic disorder that leads to an inability to execute the putt. It is in large part due to loss of confidence and concentration. Good putters think positively that they will make the putt. Although they may three putt from time to time, they do not let this bother them as they approach the next hole. I once saw a car with the automobile license plate number "Mr3putt"—this is not positive thinking. There is no perfect putter or technically correct stroke. Do what works for you. Practice making that short putt—develop confidence. Relax your approach to putting and avoid negative comments such as "I need to make this putt." You will reduce your anxiety level and improve your performance.

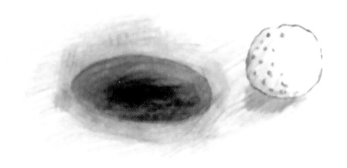

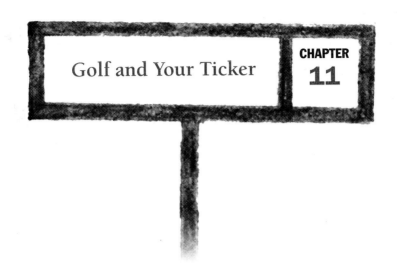

Golf and Your Ticker

Golf is like a love affair. If you take it seriously, it's no fun; if you don't take it seriously, it breaks your heart.

—Arnold Daly

The idea that one can play golf and reduce the risk of heart disease at the same time sounds too good to be true. In fact, some of us think our golf game is going to give us a stroke (no pun intended!). However, we know that golf, especially when walked, can help alter some of the risk factors associated with heart disease. A scientific study has shown that if you play golf three times a week and walk the course, you can lower your cholesterol level![1] Golf can be a healthful activity, but remember, you need to walk!

Individuals with coronary artery disease have an obstruction in the artery that supplies the heart muscle with blood. If the heart muscle does not receive enough blood and oxygen, the golfer may experience chest tightness, or arm or jaw discomfort. Activities that increase our heart rate, such as anxiety on the first tee, climbing a steep hill, or playing on hot humid days, increase the heart's need for more "fuel" (blood and oxygen). When a blockage is present, and an activity demands more blood flow to the heart muscle but this demand cannot be met, the golfer experiences the discomfort known as angina. Golfers may experience angina not only with physical stress and fatigue on the course but also with anxiety. Angry outbursts after hitting a poor shot, or the stress of making a three-foot putt in the club tournament can result in an angina episode.

Angina is the result of a temporary decrease in blood flow to the heart muscle. It dissipates when the activity or stressful situation is stopped and the requirement for additional blood flow to the heart muscle is no longer needed. Individuals with angina take nitroglycerin (NTG) tablets, placed under the tongue, for relief. NTG pills act by temporarily dilating the blood vessels, which allows more blood and oxygen to get to the heart muscle and relieves the discomfort.

A heart attack is different from angina in that blockage of the artery is 100 percent and the pain is not relieved with rest. A heart attack is a life-threatening situation that requires immediate medical treatment.

Recovering from Surgery

Many golfers who have had heart attacks, balloon angioplasties, or coronary bypass surgery have returned to the game. Some of the heroes of the sport have already proved that feat possible by their speedy return to the course following serious heart problems. Former U.S. Open and PGA champion Julius Boros underwent a quintuple bypass one year and was back to competitive golf the next—his best ever Senior Tour campaign took place the following year. Bob Rossburg, a noted professional, underwent triple bypass surgery following

Links to Experience

Chi Chi Rodriguez

The sword-dancing Chi Chi Rodriguez never considered himself a candidate for a heart attack. Blessed with a family history of longevity, his grandparents lived past the age of 100 years. For months he noticed jaw discomfort but paid it little attention. One day, after hours of what he thought was indigestion, his friends forced him to go to the hospital, where he found out he was having a heart attack. Rodriguez said, "If I would have waited another ten minutes, the doctor told me that I would have damaged my whole heart." He now says, "Don't be stubborn—if you have pain, go to the doctor."

After his heart attack in October, Rodriguez changed his diet, established an exercise routine, and gave up cigarettes. Four months after his attack, Chi Chi returned to the Senior Tour to play in the American Express Invitational.

As he reflected, "In bed when I was almost dead, I found out about life. Money doesn't mean anything. Your health is everything."

a heart attack but was back on the tour just four months later, playing in the Legends of Golf tournament.

But, you say, you aren't a hero and you're definitely not a legend. You've had a heart attack that has left you shaken and scared. Lying in bed after your own triple bypass, you wonder if you'll even be able to make it to the bathroom alone. Golf? Maybe next season.

Relax. It's perfectly normal to feel this way. Most people need a bit of time to adjust to this new image of themselves as a person with a heart problem. It shouldn't surprise you if for days, or even weeks, you cannot face the thought of getting back to your old routine. A heart attack or an invasive cardiac procedure is as much an emotional event as a physical one. Both your body and your soul will need time to heal. It may be reassuring to know, however, that your old routines are still accessible. If golf was a big part of your life before your heart attack, there is no reason it can't continue to be one.

I encourage my golfing patients, depending on their clinical condition, to begin putting and chipping as part of their cardiac rehabilitation process. Bypass patients can begin to swing a club within three to four weeks of surgery. Fears about tearing one's stitches or actually damaging the repair work done inside their hearts are as common as they are groundless. Once the healing process has begun, there is no danger of ripping open either your incision or the sutures.

It may worry you that your backswing is a little slower during the convalescent period, but think your reaction through. Many players, once they analyze the slower swing in terms of their performance, discover a decided improvement in their game. A full range of motion and a return to a normal swing (if you decide that it actually is better!) can be expected within six to eight weeks of surgery. With the advent of new procedures such as balloon angioplasty and mini coronary bypass surgery, you can be back on the links within two to three days of your procedure.

Pacemakers

Many golfers whose hearts are otherwise sound nonetheless require a pacemaker. The purpose of a pacemaker is to provide the signal to the heart to beat. People who need these battery-powered electrical devices have abnormally slow heart rates. Even a small increase in activity may make them dizzy or cause them to faint. In the past, pacemakers were set at a standard seventy beats per minute, but sophisticated new technology now makes it possible to program the pacemaker to raise the

Links **to Experience**

Bob, a fifty-two-year-old insurance executive, sat waiting for his physician, who was already fifteen minutes late for his appointment. Bob could feel himself growing increasingly irritated. The receptionist explained that the physician had been called to the hospital on an emergency and that she had been unable to reach Bob in time to reschedule his appointment. Almost in spite of himself, Bob started arguing with her, his voice getting louder and more agitated even as she tried to calm him down. Luckily, the physician arrived then and Bob was ushered into the examining room.

By the time he was undressed and the physician came in, Bob had relaxed enough to apologize. "I don't know what gets into me sometimes," he said, shaking his head ruefully. "I'm really sorry."

"Maybe you could send my receptionist some flowers," his physician suggested, smiling. "She's the one who deserves the apology." As he began the examination, he continued to make small talk, sensing that Bob was still a bit tense. "How's your handicap these days? You're still playing, aren't you?"

Bob looked pleased. "Three times a week now," he said. "I'm down to twelve."

"Well, good for you! I wish I could say that. I hope you're walking the course."

"Oh, yes" he answered, looking even more pleased. "But that reminds me of something I meant to ask you about." He then went on to describe a situation that was beginning to give him some concern. "I know you're a big advocate of walking," he said, "but lately it seems to aggravate my 'golfer's rib'. By the end of the course, I find I get a lot of muscle tension here." He spread his hand across his chest as he spoke. "Maybe the walking is too much."

"That's not very likely," the physician replied, shaking his head. "Do you get this 'muscle tension' in any other situation?"

"Well," Bob said slowly, "Now that you mention it, I do sometimes get it when I'm upset or overanxious on the course. It's the worst at the first tee, for some reason, especially if there's another group watching me tee off. And if I mess up a shot—well, you've seen what a temper I have."

His physician had heard enough. He explained to Bob that his problem was more likely to be with his heart than his 'golfer's rib' and he suggested Bob undergo a series of tests to rule out any underlying cardiac disease. An exercise stress test was all that was required to confirm his suspicions: Bob was experiencing angina, or chest pain, because of a severe coronary blockage. When he was fatigued late in a round of golf, or under stress due to performance anxiety or frustration over a poor shot, his heart required more blood and oxygen to do its work, but was unable to get it due to the blockage—hence the pain or, as he described it, "muscle tension." In Bob's case, balloon angioplasty solved the immediate problem; a low-fat diet, increased exercise and a commitment to manage stress more creatively should keep him healthy for the long run. To no one's surprise, part of Bob's overall fitness program includes golf not three, but now four times a week. And his handicap is down to ten!

Bob's experience is not an uncommon one. His nervousness at teeing off and the resulting chest pain is so common it even has a name— we call it "first tee angina." Anxiety as well as physical stress increase the demands placed on the heart. Many golfers with heart disease (recognized or unrecognized) play well during their routine rounds but develop angina during tournaments because of the heightened emotional pressure. If you experience chest pain at any time during your game, don't assume it's from walking or that it is due to the way you swing your club. See your physician. You want to go on playing golf for many years to come—don't take unnecessary chances.

heart rate automatically whenever the patient needs it. Translated to golf, that means that putting, for example, may require a heart rate of only sixty beats per minute, while climbing a steep hill carrying a golf bag may increase it to 115 beats. If you do need to get a pacemaker installed, be sure to let your physician know that you are a golfer. Since some pacemakers may be affected by muscle movement in the chest, a right-handed golfer should have the unit placed in the upper left chest area. This way, your swing will not be affected.

In spite of all the health benefits one can attain through the game, however, it must still be said that golf alone cannot provide sufficient exercise to ensure overall good health. For most people, golf is a seasonal activity and even in proper season it is governed by the weather. Finally, only those who are fortunate can afford to play golf every day, which is what you'd need to do if it were your only form of exercise. Ultimately, golf must be seen as a complementary exercise, with the added bonus that whatever else you do to improve your general fitness, it can only improve your handicap.

> *It's not your life, it's not your wife, it's only a game.*
>
> Lloyd Mangrum

Guidelines for the Cardiac Golfer

Playing in Warm Weather

In hot weather, the heart works harder and faster to supply the skin with a greater flow of blood to keep the body cool. This results in an increased demand on the heart muscle.

- Try to avoid playing golf on hot, humid days. It is best in these conditions to play early in the morning or during the evening hours.
- Try to avoid prolonged periods of exposure to sunlight.

Playing in Cold Weather

Cold temperatures cause the body's blood vessels to constrict, resulting in higher blood pressure, and putting additional demands on the heart.

- Avoid playing golf in the cold early mornings and go out when the sun is the warmest: between the hours of 10:00 A.M. and 2:00 P.M.
- Dress appropriately for cool or cold weather by layering clothing and wearing a hat and gloves.

When to Call Your Doctor

If you have a heart condition, any change in the frequency, location, severity, or intensity of angina should be reported. Angina is that chest or arm discomfort that may be perceived as a pressure, tightness, squeezing, burning, or aching. It may also occur in the throat or jaw.

- If these discomforts are accompanied by sweating and nausea, notify your physician.
- It is important to be aware that stress, as well as physical exertion, can precipitate angina. Stress can be brought on by the sudden onset of angina or frustration after a poorly hit shot. Often a golfer will become angry or impatient while waiting for the group ahead to hit or putt out.
- Because club tournament play increases our anxiety level, it may precipitate an episode of angina.
- In addition to chest pain, severe shortness of breath while playing golf may be a sign of a cardiovascular problem that requires treatment.

Other Causes of Chest Pain

Inflammation of the chest wall muscles, bursitis, arthritis, and even indigestion, can produce symptoms that parallel those associated with angina. Often the golfer attributes his or her discomfort to muscle strain from poor swing mechanics. Golfer's rib, or musculoskeletal pain, occurs primarily with deep breathing, bending, turning, and swinging a club. It will not be relieved with nitroglycerin (NTG). Nevertheless, if you have chest discomfort, don't assume it is one of these medical conditions or a problem with your swing. Instead, consult your physician as well as your golf pro.

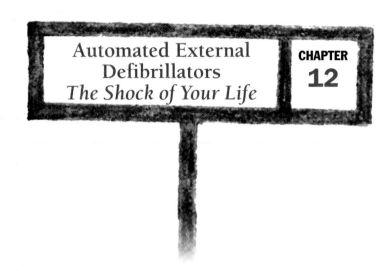

Automated External Defibrillators
The Shock of Your Life

I'm learning to take the bad days better. This isn't a matter of life and death.

—Dottie Pepper

More than 250,000 people in the United States die each year from cardiac arrest before they reach a hospital. Cardiac arrest, a complication arising from a heart attack, can cause a person to collapse within seconds. The fifth likeliest public location in the United States at which to collapse from a sudden cardiac arrest is the golf course.[4] It is not the golf itself that leads to this astounding statistic, but rather the age of the average golfer, and the time spent playing the sport.

Currently, fewer than five percent of cardiac arrest victims survive. The key to saving lives from sudden cardiac arrest is early recognition of the problem and activation of the EMS system, early CPR, early defibrillation, and early advanced life support. These four elements act as links in a chain, and comprise the American Heart Association's "Chain of Survival" for cardiac arrest. When these links work together, a person's chance of survival is greatly increased.

CPR keeps oxygen-rich blood flowing to the brain and heart after a cardiac arrest. Early defibrillation can now be done with a new life-saving device, the automated external defibrillator (AED). An AED is a portable, computerized defibrillator that can deliver an electric current, or shock, to a heart that has gone into an abnormal electrical rhythm.

A heart attack victim's chance of survival decreases
approximately 10% for each minute without treatment.

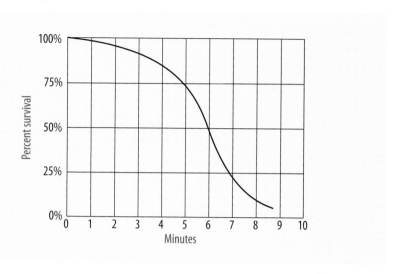

The AED contains a cardiac rhythm analysis system that decides whether the heart needs to be shocked. The device walks you through the simple steps of the defibrillation process. All you need to do is turn it on and follow the voice prompts, which direct you to place pads attached to the AED on the person's chest, and press the buttons the AED directs you to press, at the times it directs you to do so. If a shock is needed, the AED charges to a preset energy level. The shock it delivers very briefly stops the heart, which allows it to resume its normal rhythm. If a shock is not needed, the AED will tell you so.

Just because a shock is not indicated does not mean the person is OK. In some cases, it simply means that the specific rhythm that responds to defibrillation is not present. If the person is still pulseless, then he or she is still in cardiac arrest. CPR is needed until EMS personnel arrive.

AEDs weigh only a few pounds, and are battery-powered. They are relatively inexpensive and need little maintenance. AEDs are easily used by anyone, and are beginning to be stored in many public and private places, including the pro shops of golf courses. At the same time, responding to the endorsement

by the American Heart Association of public access defibrillation as a national initiative, many laypeople such as security guards, lifeguards, and maintenance personnel, are being trained to use AEDs.

If you have a heart condition, or know that one of your fellow golfers has a heart condition, check with your pro shop to see if the course you are playing has an AED on the premises. If someone collapses on the course, you should still call 911 or your local emergency number so professional help can arrive as quickly as possible, but until they arrive, you can make the difference between a person's surviving a cardiac arrest and not surviving.

Lobby your club or home course to purchase an AED and have personnel trained in its use, as well as CPR. You can even learn how to use one yourself by taking a course from the National Safety Council or the American Heart Association.

Health Tip: Learn to recognize the signs of a heart attack. If you find yourself suffering from shortness of breath, chest, arm, neck, or jaw pain, seek immediate medical care. Don't wait until you're stricken by cardiac arrest. Stop one before it happens.

Links *to Experience*

At age fifty-six, Jack Van Houten was living in Houston, Texas, where he managed to play a round of golf about once a week. Every Saturday, he and his buddies would have a friendly competitive match. During one match, after hitting his tee shot on seventeen, Jack recalls "the last thing I remember is being dizzy and falling to the ground." Jack was in cardiac arrest. In the group following them was a young man who had just completed a CPR course the prior evening. He, along with his fellow players, administered CPR. A marshal driving by radioed the pro shop. Immediately other personnel arrived and Jack was "shocked" back to life with a defibrillator. Jack said, "I was really lucky to have people around me who knew CPR, a marshal to summon help, and a defibrillator to save me." Today Jack Van Houten takes medication, has a permanent implantable defibrillator, and plays golf three times a week.

Use of an AED on a golf course

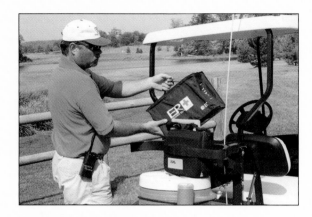

A golf course employee loads an emergency response bag and the AED onto the ER cart for the day.

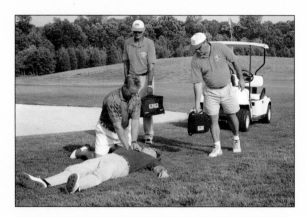

Golf staff arrive to help an apparent heart attack victim.

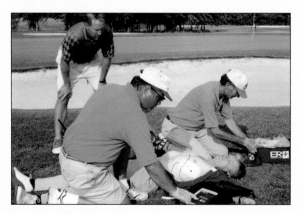

Emergency personnel activate an AED.

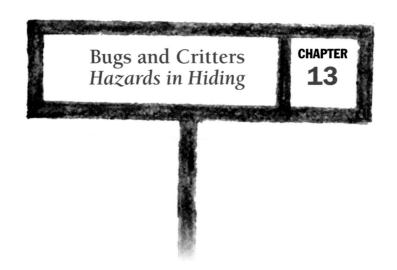

Bugs and Critters
Hazards in Hiding

CHAPTER 13

One of the beauties of golf is the natural environment in which it is played. The shape of the land determines the layout of the course. It follows, therefore, that every golf course in the world is different, and that each one has its unique delights and its own special hazards. It also follows, much though we may hate to admit it, that many factors affecting the game are beyond our control. The ocean breezes at Pebble Beach in California cannot be quelled, no matter how difficult they make it to concentrate, nor is it possible to avoid the Swilcan Burn water hazard at St. Andrews in Scotland, frustrating though it may be, especially to the inexperienced golfer.

Similarly, though many attempts have been made, we as a race have been unsuccessful in subduing the world of insects and microbes. The highest paid business executives will still howl in pain when stung by a bee and the most important politician can still be humbled by the deer tick who carries Lyme disease. The point is that in playing golf we are confronting the natural world—the possibility of making the acquaintance of insects we'd rather not get to know is a strong one. It helps to be prepared. First aid for bug and critter encounters is covered in Chapter 21.

Lyme Disease

Lyme disease is by now a fairly well-known disease, which means that if you do come down with it, it will most likely be diagnosed early on—unlike the situation in the early 1980s when physicians across the country were mystified by a condition they could not recognize. Although it was first identified back in 1975 by Dr. Allen Steere in Lyme, Connecticut, it wasn't until the late 1980s that a widespread incidence of the disease was noted. Subsequent coverage in the popular press made it more familiar to nonmedical people as well.

Lyme disease is spread by a tick so minute it can barely be seen. The tick is carried by deer and white-footed mice. Its favored habitat is any wooded area, but tall grasses and brush are also favorite hiding spots for this critter. If you are like most golfers (myself included), this is an area you know all too well. In other words, if your ball goes anywhere but right down the middle of the fairway, you are at risk. The risk is even higher for golf course personnel whose job involves maintenance of the grounds because, for them, avoiding the rough is not an option.

If you don't notice that you have been bitten (which is very likely), early symptoms are confusing and unpredictable. Of those infected with the disease, seventy-five percent develop a typical red rash at the site of the bite. This rash is described in the literature as a "bull's-eye" rash because its expanding round shape encircles a small welt at its center. In some cases, this rash is the first and last sign you will get of having the disease. It clears up in a few days and you may never even associate it with Lyme disease.

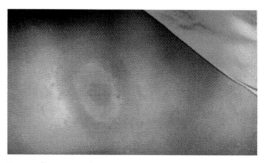

Lyme disease rash

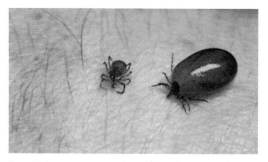

Deer ticks; not engorged and blood-engorged

In other cases, however, the rash is just the beginning. Flu-like symptoms then develop, with patients suffering fever, fatigue, chills, headaches, and pain in the joints. If the disease is detected right then, and treated immediately with antibiotics, chances are good that it will be eliminated. But the disease has been known to drag on, and even progress into more serious disabilities like arthritis, heart problems, facial paralysis, and severe headaches. It is important, therefore, to get treatment if you suspect you have been bitten. A blood test gives a reliable reading between two and four weeks after the bite.

Like most other diseases, prevention is much more effective than trying to cure it once it is an accomplished fact. During the tick's prime season, July through September, and particularly in the northeast and central states or Pacific Coast, protect yourself by dressing appropriately. Long sleeves and long pants (tucked into your socks is ideal if you've got the nerve!) are your best bet, and spraying your clothing (not your skin) with a tick repellent will also help. Permethrin (Permanone) is an extremely potent insecticide that works both to kill and repel ticks. A one-minute application to the outside of your pants and shirt/jacket can give almost 100 percent protection. A vaccine called Lymerix, recently developed by Smith Kline Beecham, can be effective in preventing Lyme disease. The three inoculations are given over a twelve-month period and will result in immunity for eighty percent of golfers.

The moment the tick burrows into your skin is not the moment it begins its task of infecting you. You have twenty-four hours to remove this little time bomb before it explodes, so it is worth the effort of checking your skin carefully after playing golf to be sure you have no uninvited guests.

If you do find one, use tweezers to grasp it firmly behind its head and pull slowly and steadily. If you squeeze its body, you may end up forcing the Lyme disease bacterium into your own body. Once the tick is out, wash your hands and the wound site, and apply antiseptic. Keep watching for a rash (remember it can appear as long as eight weeks after the event). If you do get one, consult your physician.

LYME DISEASE: WHAT YOU SHOULD KNOW

WHAT TO LOOK FOR

- Fatigue and malaise
- Headache
- Stiff neck
- Muscle aches
- Fever
- A red rash often in shape of a bull's eye occurring within thirty days of bite
- Flu-like symptoms in first month
- Arthritis and fatigue that develop after four months

PREVENTION: WHAT TO DO

- Wear long pants tucked into socks if walking in woods or tall grass.
- Spray exposed skin with tick repellent.
- Treat clothing with repellent that contains permethrin.
- Ask your physician about the Lymerix vaccine.

Two other diseases transmitted by ticks are Rocky Mountain spotted fever and Ehrlichiosis. Rocky Mountain spotted fever is now more prevalent in the southern and eastern states than it is in the mountain states. The majority of cases occur in May, June, and July. The symptoms include a high fever, chills, headache, muscle aches, abdominal pain, nausea, and a characteristic spotted rash. Usually, the rash first develops on the wrists, hands, and ankles several days after the bite. Ehrlichiosis is less common and can be confused with the flu. The symptoms include a high fever, headache, chills, muscle aches, and loss of appetite. A distinguishing symptom is extreme sensitivity to light. Most cases occur in south central and southern Atlantic states, but it might be on the rise in the central states such as Indiana. Both Rocky Mountain spotted fever and Ehrlichiosis are treated with antibiotics.

Fire Ants

Fire ants are another natural hazard of the golf course. Although they are limited presently to the southeastern part of the country, especially Florida, they have been seen as far west as Texas and they seem determined to, one day, make it to California. Fire ants are extremely aggressive creatures who will attack, in swarms of thousands, any moving object that they perceive as a threat to their mounded homes. As a rule, fire ants are not found on the open fairways because of the constant mowing and the regular applications of chemical fertilizers and pesticides. In the rough where they feel safe, however, they may cause serious problems for golfers.

The sting of the fire ant is particularly painful because one ant will sting repeatedly in the same spot. The venom thus introduced into the body of the victim creates a burning, painful sensation at the site, hence the name "fire ants." The symptoms and signs generally subside within minutes to hours. With thousands of ants attacking at the same time, the victim generally suffers multiple stings, so that the aftermath is extremely painful and occasionally life threatening. An allergy to fire ant venom may result in anaphylactic shock. Warning signs include severe swelling in parts of the body that were not stung, such as the eyes, lips, and tongue. Additional symptoms include severe itching, anxiety, nausea, vomiting, coughing, difficult breathing, fainting, unconsciousness, and the sudden appearance of hives all over the body. Anaphylactic reactions require emergency medical treatment. Call 911 or your local emergency number as soon as you get stung. Deaths have been associated with fire ant bites so it's important to take immediate action.

Avoiding the fire ant is easier than avoiding the deer tick. Like most insects, fire ants attack only when they believe their mounds are threatened.

If your course is located in a geographic area known to have fire ants, it is important to educate yourself, and especially your unknowing guests, about the presence of fire ants. Encourage your home course to post signs to alert players to the presence of fire ants along with instructions not to disturb the fire ants' mound. (See Chapter 21 for important first aid information.)

Fire Ant Distribution in the United States

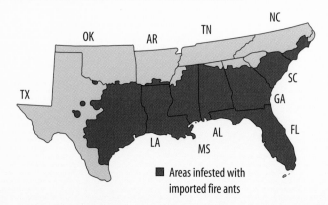

Areas infested with imported fire ants

Bee Stings

Bees, wasps, and ants use their weapons to protect themselves. Most do so in a predictable manner, but others, like the ground-nesting yellow jackets are aggressive and may attack without provocation. Yellow jackets can also inflict multiple stings. Wasps and yellow jackets are attracted to food and garbage containers so it's important to dispense of that soda can!

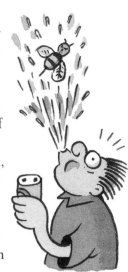

The African bee, a fierce new strain of the insect which, some years ago, arrived in this country via Brazil presents yet another problem to golfers. Like the fire ant, this so-called killer bee is fanatic about protecting its hive. An unluckily aimed golf ball or a careless jostling of bushes in the rough may disturb a hive and alarm its inhabitants, who will then attack in a merciless wave.

Most bee stings result in a painful raised hive caused by the venom. The site becomes red, swollen, and itchy. The first step in treatment is to remove any retained stinger. Ice should be applied to the site, along with mild analgesics if necessary. The most severe reaction to a bee sting is anaphylaxis, which is a life-threatening emergency that requires immediate medical attention. Golfers who have known allergic reactions to bee stings should carry self-injectable epinephrine in their golf bag and inform their playing partners of its location prior to play.

Spider Bites

The bite of most spiders causes little or no reaction. If symptoms do occur, they are local and can be treated with ice packs or analgesics. The brown recluse spider (or fiddleback) is found in the Midwest and south central region of the United States. The reaction to their bite is generally local but occasionally causes a systemic reaction. The reaction is red with purple discoloration at the site and the center becomes black when the tissue dies. Treatment is with analgesics and ice. A physician should be consulted for possible antibiotic use.

The bite of a black widow spider results in immediate pain and local reaction. Initial treatment should include the application of ice and elevation at the site of the bite. This is an emergency and you should call 911 or your local emergency number.

Geographic Location of Snakes in the United States

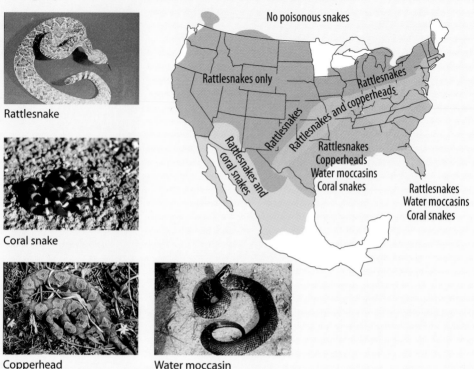

Rattlesnake

Coral snake

Copperhead

Water moccasin

No poisonous snakes

Rattlesnakes only

Rattlesnakes and copperheads

Rattlesnakes and coral snakes

Rattlesnakes
Copperheads
Water moccasins
Coral snakes

Rattlesnakes
Water moccasins
Coral snakes

Snake Bites

In the United States, the rattlesnake, coral snake, copperhead, and cotton mouth are poisonous snakes of concern to the golfer. Coral snakes are about two feet long with yellow-red-yellow-black bands. The familiar saying "Red and black, friend of Jack. Red and yellow, kill a fellow" refers to the coral snake. Most snake bites occur in the Southeast. Should a player get bitten, place a constrictor band a few inches above the bite, and immobilize the extremity. Call 911 or your local emergency number for help, and do not let the golfer walk back to the clubhouse. (See Chapter 21 for emergency treatment procedures.)

Before you put anything in your mouth, think about where it has been!

Pesticides and Chemicals

It is important to consider a health issue often overlooked by golfers: the golf course itself. That gorgeous rolling expanse of grass didn't appear by magic, nor can it be maintained that way. To achieve the kind of quality turf we expect and to eliminate the bugs and critters we detest require enormous effort, constant attention, tremendous amounts of water, and large doses of chemical fertilizers and pesticides. The environmental issues involved in this level of maintenance affect our health both directly and indirectly. The chemicals used are toxic to all who are exposed to this environment. Pesticides, which in some countries may contain mercury for treatment of fungi, are usually sprayed in the morning. Fungicides are primarily applied to tees and greens, and generally there is little runoff into the environment. These chemicals are most active when wet, and require approximately two to three hours to dry. The grass, thatch, and soil absorb most of the chemicals. Golfers with early morning tee times need to be especially concerned about direct contamination of the skin from contact with tainted balls or tees. If you can see the blue-green tracer dye before you play, consider the fungicide active and defer your tee time.

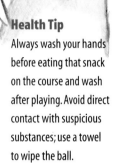

Health Tip
Always wash your hands before eating that snack on the course and wash after playing. Avoid direct contact with suspicious substances; use a towel to wipe the ball.

Many courses are irrigated with wastewater from sewage treatment plants. Chewing on a tee is inoculating oneself with bacteria, pesticides, and fungicides.

Although fewer players are smoking cigarettes on the course, cigar smoking is on the rise. Putting a cigar in your mouth after picking it up off the tee or green is very likely to introduce pesticides into your body. Contamination can result in illnesses ranging from minor skin rashes, nausea, and vomiting to severe respiratory symptoms and possibly cancer.

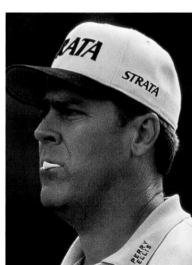

Hal Sutton

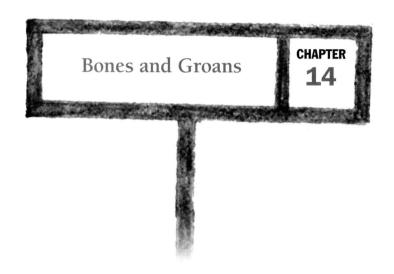

Bones and Groans

CHAPTER 14

If your adversary is a hole or two down, there is no serious cause for alarm in his complaining of a severely sprained wrist, or an acute pain, resembling lumbago, which checks his swing. Should he happen to win the next hole, these symptoms will in all probability become less troublesome.

—Horace Hutchinson

It is reported that in the 1920s, a father sustained a mortal blow to the head from his frustrated son to whom he was giving a golf lesson. The moral here is, let your PGA Professional teach your family. Assaults with clubs aside, many golfers are plagued by injuries. It is not surprising that, given the variations in swing mechanics and frequency of play and ability, there is a variety of injury patterns. Injuries vary from blisters, caused by hitting too many balls early in the season, to problems with the back or shoulder that may require surgery.

Most golf injuries are due to the pressures extensive play puts on the body. Tour professionals, for example, average two injuries per year and, like those of amateurs, they are generally due to extra strain of the

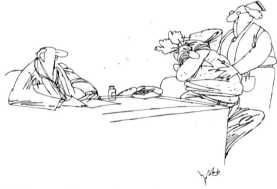

"This happened to you after you hit your longest drive? Well, that's some consolation."

muscles. Fred Couples, Jack Nicklaus, and Payne Stewart continue to deal with their chronic back problems. Nancy Lopez wears a knee brace because of cartilage loss in her knees.

The player with a high handicap compounds the risk of injury with poor swing mechanics. These players tend to generate more power or club head speed by using their arms, whereas the professional has the correct body weight shift, generating power in the hips and legs. For both the amateur and the professional, the back is the most frequent site of injury. Again, because of swing mechanics, the less talented golfer is likely to put more stress on the lumbar spine. Don't be surprised when you try to "kill" that three-wood shot to reach a distant green and you feel a sharp pull in your back—acute muscle strain!

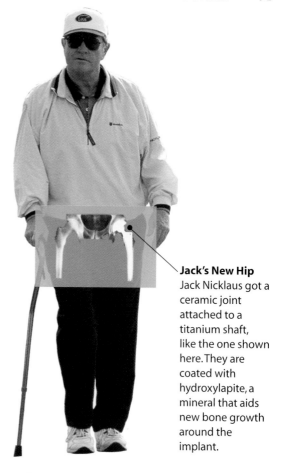

Jack's New Hip
Jack Nicklaus got a ceramic joint attached to a titanium shaft, like the one shown here. They are coated with hydroxylapite, a mineral that aids new bone growth around the implant.

Golfer's elbow is a form of tendonitis that has affected golfers for generations. It results when a muscle is irritated or torn. Although generally the result of the muscle's overuse, it may occur acutely when the club head comes to an abrupt stop after hitting a rock or root, or from practicing off a hard rubber mat. With the abrupt stop comes the tearing of the muscle. For most golfers, it is the left or lead elbow, while in tennis players, the tendonitis most often affects the right elbow. Men and women are affected equally by this problem. Although men have more back problems, the risk of wrist injury appears more frequently in women. The shoulder, ribs, and feet are not immune to overuse injury. Some of you may even be aware of overuse injury to the foot by opponents who assist the ball back into the fairway.

Seniors and Injury

Golfers over the age of fifty comprise twenty-five percent of the golfing population, but account for nearly fifty percent of all rounds played. It is not surprising that those of us who love the sport and have more time than young career-builders tend to play more. Our handicaps may not go down but our risk of injury certainly goes up.

Whether you are fifty or eighty years old, the most common cause of injuries is overuse. As we get older and leave the world of the "flat bellies," changes occur in our body and physiology. Cartilage begins to lose water and may become brittle, and crack more easily. It takes less force to tear this cartilage in senior players than in the younger individual with "rubbery cartilage." If we have been active most of our lives, then wear and tear on our knee cartilage can occur at an earlier age. Nancy Lopez, who has had an outstanding career on the LPGA Tour, now must wear a knee brace. She is considering surgical options including arthroscopic surgery.

Health Tip
Prevention of injuries begins in the off-season with conditioning programs and strengthening of muscles of the back, shoulder, wrist, and abdomen.

Osteoporosis is another common problem that faces the golfer with age. This process results in a thinning or weakening of the bones. It may account for compression fracture in the back or vertebrae (we are not as tall as we once were). Although osteoporosis may result in some back pain, there is no reason to discontinue playing. Mild exercise, in fact, retards bone loss. To reduce the effects of osteoporosis, get out and play golf. Just remember, you need to walk.

Playing with Arthritis

Although arthritis can occur at any age, it generally begins after age forty and is termed osteoarthritis. This process affects the cartilage of the hips, knees, and back, as well as the hands. Bob Murphy, who currently excels on the Senior Tour, nearly had to give up the game because of this problem. The golfer may experience pain or stiffness, especially with an early morning tee time. The discomfort of aches and pains may last thirty minutes but in the severe type known as rheumatoid arthritis, discomforts can last up to hours at a time. Most golfers with this condition can play safely and regularly without damaging the joints. Pain can be managed with anti-inflammatory agents such as aspirin or with prescription drugs, which may have a stronger anti-inflammatory effect. Analgesics may prove helpful if taken prior to the round. For Bob Murphy, strong anti-inflammatory agents were necessary to manage his arthritis, and they did enable him to return to the top of the Senior Tour.

For the golfer, the best treatment for arthritis is a combination of exercise and medication. If arthritis is affecting your game, consider doing flexibility exercises before playing. Changing your equipment including balls, shafts, grips, and shoes will also be helpful.

Equipment

Shafts are available with graphite and lightweight steel. The lighter club promotes increased club-head speed and distance. Graphite has the capacity to absorb the shock of impact. Lanny Watkins switched to heavy graphite to avoid the aches and pains he got in his hands and elbows. Distance can be increased as well by extending the length of the driver, which creates a bigger arc. Perimeter-weighted clubs are better for shock absorption from off-center hits. Try using a lower compression ball, ninety or even eighty compression; it will feel softer when hit and distance will be unaffected.

In addition to weight, the senior player should consider the flexibility of the shaft. The location of the flex, or kickpoint, of the shaft will determine the flight of the ball. A shaft with a low kickpoint (more flex near the head) will launch the ball at a higher angle—get it airborne. After years of playing, I've discovered that air offers less resistance than grass.

Arthritis in Your Hands

If arthritis affects your hands, adjustments can be made to improve your swing. You can also try a flexibility exercise simply by stretching out the fingers and bringing them into the palm. Arthritic conditions may limit the ability to maintain a strong grip, which results in your twisting the club at impact. You can choose grips to overcome this problem. A mid-size or jumbo grip may feel more comfortable if arthritis is the problem. Grip size however will affect the flight of the ball and should be adjusted to suit the size and condition of the golfer's hands. A small grip will promote more hand action and tend to result in a draw or pull. A larger grip will restrict hand action and promote a fade or push. The use of an air-cushion-type grip incorporates some air chambers into the core of the grip. This produces a soft comfortable feel that has the ability to absorb the shock of a mis-hit.

Aching Back

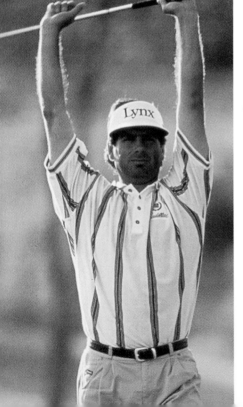

Senior Tour player George Archer is familiar with injuries. During his twenty-seven year career he has had surgery on his wrist, shoulder, and back. Despite playing with steel rods inserted in his back eighteen years ago, he remains competitive on tour.

Health Tip

That back pain you have might be a stress fracture in the back caused by overswinging.

Back injuries are common and affect ninety percent of the general population. For the golfer, professional and amateur alike, the back remains the most common area of injury. Notable PGA players Jack Nicklaus, Payne Stewart, and Bernard Langer have suffered from this affliction. Injuries to the back may be the result of muscle strains, herniated discs, and even arthritis. The vast majority of these injuries are due to overuse in combination with poor swing mechanics.

The golf swing is responsible for wear-and-tear injuries of our lumbar region as a result of the forward flexion in the spine during swing rotation. Excessive practice at the range may result in strains and sprains of the muscles and the ligaments in the lower back. Most of these injuries will heal with rest and heat. Poor conditioning and fatigue predispose the golfer to injury. If we can't hold the trunk rigid throughout our swing, it may increase the lateral forces and stress on the back, resulting in injury.

Poor swing mechanics can lead to excessive flexion in the back, which causes strain and pain. Even the professional who uses the same basic well-grooved swing with the same muscles for each shot is subjected to problems with his or her back. Tiger Woods has a huge swing coil that requires considerable flexibility, and he's already starting to have back pain. It will be interesting to see if he can avoid serious problems as he gets older. Amateurs, like myself, who have very unpredictable and inconsistent swings, are at risk for more frequent injuries. Seeking counsel from our local professional may not enable us to join the tour but may help us avoid that pain in the back.

Fred Couples

PREVENTION AND TREATMENT OF BACK INJURY: WHAT YOU SHOULD KNOW

- Start when removing your bag from the car—bring your bag and clubs close to the edge of the trunk and bend your knees as you lift out the bag.
- If your back hurts on one side, carry it on the good side or use a pull cart.
- Even if you don't have problems with your back, consider switching to a double strap that equally distributes the weight of the bag.
- If you do carry your bag, make sure it has a stand.
- Bend your knees when picking up or placing the ball on the tee.
- If you're overweight, you contribute to increased stress to the back. Studies show that each pound you lose from the upper body removes three to four pounds of stress from your back.
- Control of the trunk is easier if you develop a more compact swing. This can be accomplished by reducing both your backswing and follow-through.
- When putting, bend the knees slightly to avoid excessive bending at the waist. Some golfers have gone to the extra-long putter to reduce discomfort and improve mechanics.
- Avoid carts. Sitting is one of the worst positions for back strain. When sitting in a cart, our muscles cool down. We then jump out of the cart and hit a ball with a full swing likely to produce injury. Try walking the course, which will keep the muscles warmed up throughout the round.
- With back problems, stretching, strengthening, and flexibility exercises are essential.

Exercises for the Back

When you begin a new exercise program, do as many repetitions as you can without pain. Increase the holding times and repetitions as you get more comfortable with the routines. And check with your physician before starting any exercise regime.

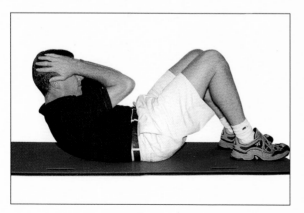

1. Curl-ups Lie on your back and bend your knees. Put your hands beside your ears. Do not clasp your hands behind your neck. Curl up until your shoulder blades are off the floor, then roll down to starting position.

Exercises for the Back, continued

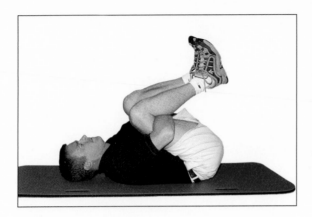

2. Double-knee bend Lie on your back with your legs flat on the floor. Clasp your hands behind your thighs and bring both legs up toward your chest. Hold for 5 to 10 seconds, breathe normally, return to starting position, rest, and repeat.

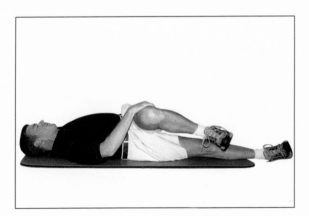

3. Back rotation Bring one knee up and slowly pull it across your hip. Keep your back as flat against the floor as possible. Hold for 5 to 10 seconds, breathe normally, return to starting position, and rest. Switch to the other knee.

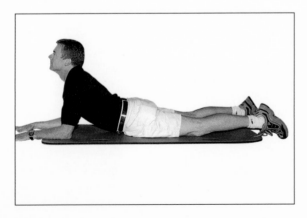

4. Back stretch Begin by lying on the floor. Lift as high as is comfortable. Hold for 5 to 10 seconds, breathe normally, return to starting position, rest, and repeat.

The Shoulder

Shoulder injuries occur more frequently in the older golfer. It is the left side that is affected in the right-handed golfer. As we approach the age of thirty-five the degenerative process begins in the shoulder. With a diminished blood supply and degenerative changes, rotator cuff function decreases. Overuse, by both the professional and amateur, results in tiny muscle tears that are responsible for the painful injury. Professional golfers may perform 2000 swings per week and suffer injury, as was the case for Beth Daniel. The likes of Keith Clearwater, Mark Calcavecchia, and Jerry Pate have had injuries to their rotator cuffs. Greg Norman recently underwent surgery to remove spurs causing inflammation in this area. Although always an option, surgery can be deferred while an attempt to alter swing mechanics is tried. Stress to the shoulder can be reduced by shortening the backswing.

> *Man, the worst thing about this is I won't be able to play golf.*
>
> Charles Barkley on his shoulder injury

We play golf for life and, since most injuries are due to hitting the ball too many times and degeneration, it is important to avoid excess practice and recognize the signs of taking too many shots on the course.

SHOULDER INJURIES: WHAT YOU SHOULD KNOW

- Immediate treatment depends on the diagnosis but will include restricted practice and playing, the application of ice, and compression.
- Rehabilitation with physical therapy may be necessary.

Strengthening Exercises for the Shoulder

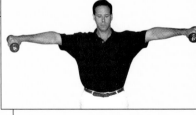

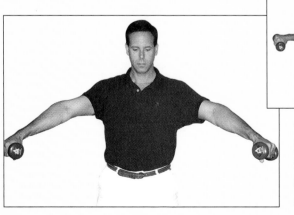

1. Rotator cuff With a weight in each hand, hold arms out and forward of your body about 30 degrees with thumb knuckles turned toward floor. Slowly raise arms to just shoulder height (insert). Return to starting position, and repeat.

Exercises for the Shoulder, continued

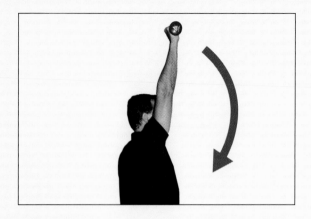

2. Rotator cuff Slowly lift the weight in front of your body and overhead. Slowly return to starting position and repeat.

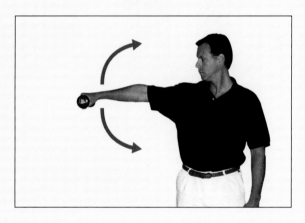

3. Rotator cuff Slowly lift the weight out to the side and overhead. As you lift, turn the hand until the palm faces your head. Slowly return to starting position and repeat.

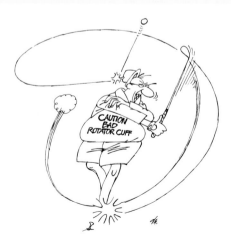

The Elbow

In the high-tech world of golf, we are armed with humongous club heads, space-age shafts, and complex contraptions to alter our swing plane, yet our bodies are required to generate the force necessary to beat those balls at the range. Those of us who are lacking that picture-perfect swing, totally in balance, place excessive stress on our joints and muscles.

The elbow is a frequent site of injury, with the left side more common in the right-handed golfer. Calvin Peete, who played on the PGA Tour, had chronic elbow problems. Golfer's elbow, or tendonitis, is the result of trauma to the muscle or tendon. These microscopic tears result in inflammation and pain. Tendonitis frequently results from the muscle's overuse (I knew I shouldn't four putt), causing many small tears in the muscle fibers. Tendonitis is Nature's way of telling you that a muscle is tired of being jerked around. If the inflammation is limited, we may be able to play with minor pain for weeks to months. Never relinquishing the opportunity to play, we continue to aggravate the condition and healing fails to occur.

We experience golfer's elbow initially as a minor twinge, which ultimately leads to pain for a period of weeks to months. The discomfort can increase to the point that it is difficult to even shake hands or pull a club from the bag. The best treatment is rest in combination with anti-inflammatory agents such as ibuprofen or aspirin. For an acute episode, an ice pack can be used to reduce the immediate periods of discomfort. Steroid injections and even surgery for severe cases have been recommended. Dana Quigley on the Senior Tour uses a strap to minimize discomfort. Although exercise offers benefits to the golfer with a painful elbow, rest remains the best form of treatment, because healing requires three to six weeks. Playing with golfer's elbow is like driving with a flat tire: although you can do it, it's hell on the equipment.

GOLFER'S ELBOW: WHAT TO DO

- Treat immediately with rest.
- Apply ice.
- Take anti-inflammatories, including nonsteroidal anti-inflammatory agents.
- Avoid excess stress to the elbow by not trying to "kill" the ball.

Exercises for Golfer's Elbow

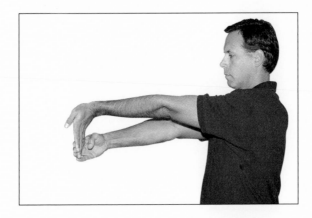

1. Stretches for golfer's elbow Gently pull hand toward you. Hold for 20 seconds, relax, and repeat for several minutes.

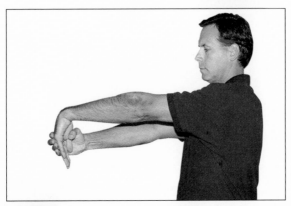

2. Stretches for golfer's elbow Gently pull hand toward you. Hold for 20 seconds, relax, and repeat for several minutes.

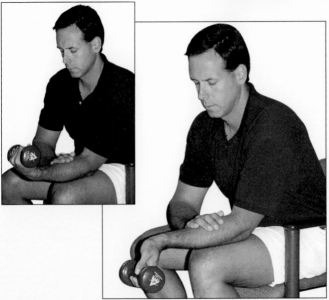

3. Strengthening for golfer's elbow Use very light weights. Curl hand up. Hold for 10 seconds, and return to starting position. Repeat three times.

Exercises for Golfer's Elbow, continued

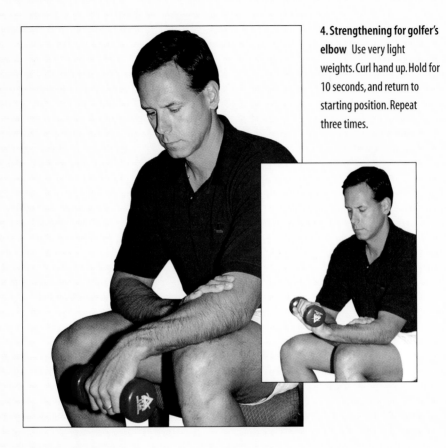

4. Strengthening for golfer's elbow Use very light weights. Curl hand up. Hold for 10 seconds, and return to starting position. Repeat three times.

The Hand and Wrist

Correct hand action is essential for proper shot execution. If distance is becoming a problem or if you lose a club at the top of the swing, the reason may be in the palm of your hand! Many wrist injuries are due to a strong grip (the left hand is rotated more to the right on the club) and holding the club too tightly.

Carpal Tunnel Syndrome

Some golfers experience numbness or pins-and-needle sensation in their hands. Nothing seems to relieve the numbness in the fingertips, which lasts twenty to thirty minutes. Often the golfer shakes his hands, trying to get life back into them. This condition is called carpal tunnel syndrome and results from nerve compression. Hitting too many buckets of balls daily or other frequent repetitive wrist motion can produce this problem. The discomfort in the fingers and wrist can occur while swinging the club, or even while at rest. Former U.S. Open champion Ken Venturi developed carpal tunnel syndrome in both hands, which ultimately ended his professional career. For most golfers, carpal tunnel syndrome can be treated with splints, anti-inflammatory agents, and in some cases, surgery. The primary problem is overuse—avoid the range and spend more time on the putting green, without having the wrist breakdown! Proper warm-up and swing mechanics prevent recurrent injury.

Tendonitis in the Wrist and Hand

Tendonitis in the wrist and hand typically develops from one mis-aimed shot. The golfer hits a tree root or a rock, usually on the downswing, and suddenly tears the tendon or muscle. These acute injuries more frequently occur in the lead left wrist and hand. This problem is generally self-limited and can be treated with rest and anti-inflammatory agents. The most common site of injury for the LPGA professional is the wrist.

A driving range in Japan

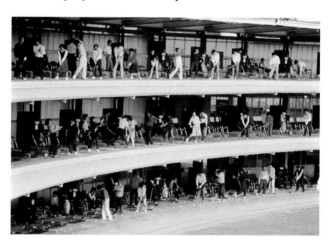

Some golfers develop tendonitis at the base of the thumb. It is often the left thumb in right-handed golfers. Again treatment requires rest and anti-inflammatory drugs. If pain in the hand is interfering with your game, you may wish to consult your physician as well as your pro (to correct your hand action).

Fractures due to golf are rare unless of course you have tripped in an animal hole, fallen out of the cart, or hit your fist in anger against an immovable object, as José María Olazabal did in the 1999 U.S. Open, forcing him to withdraw. Kerri Webb, LPGA professional, played at her first appearance at Qualifying School with a fractured wrist.

The hand is subject to an unusual fracture in golf when swinging the club and hitting a hard object; the force of the impact is transmitted to the butt end of the club, which can break one of the bones in the hand.

WRIST AND HAND INJURIES: WHAT TO DO

- If you have carpal tunnel syndrome, get rest and use splints and anti-inflammatory agents.
- For tendonitis, rest and take anti-inflammatory agents.
- Avoid hitting off tree roots and hard rubber mats.
- Consider taking medication prior to your round.

Links *to Experience*

In a world where life is sometimes stranger than fiction, one of my patients, a forty-two-year-old golf enthusiast who plays in New England, felt that his ball wouldn't carry as far in cold temperatures. Routinely, he would place the ball in his pocket, keeping it warm prior to teeing off at the next hole. Feeling this strategy was successful, he began to microwave the ball prior to going off to the first tee. This gentleman called me after one "nuking" session. He had prematurely touched the ball in the microwave oven, upon which it exploded in his hand, resulting in significant muscle and tissue damage.

The Legs

If you have taken my advice and switched from using a cart to walking, those first few rounds may have identified some muscles you didn't know you had. You may not realize the body has more than 400 muscles. After a few rounds on a hilly course, you might have thought that all those muscles are in your legs! If you have just started walking the course, it is not unusual that your muscle soreness appears to be more severe the following day. The phenomenon of delayed onset muscle soreness (DOMS) generally begins the day following exercise. It will last approximately two to three days before it subsides. A muscle is composed of many fibers that function by both contraction and relaxation. Muscles that are unaccustomed to climbing in and out of bunkers or up and down hills may experience very minute tears. As the result of this minor trauma to the muscles, tension and tightness occur, which decrease one's flexibility. We feel this diminished flexibility as soreness and pain.

Health Tip

Knee pain in golfers tends to occur when we use longer clubs. If you have pain in the knee, reduce your amount of play and use shorter irons.

If this occurs after an attempt to get more exercise from your golf by initiating a walking program, you may be questioning the logic of your decision. Don't despair, help is available. Believe it or not, this muscle soreness can be helped with mild exercise, such as walking, or even light stretching. Topical analgesics, such as Bengay®, may provide some minor relief. Not surprisingly, prevention is the best therapy and can be accomplished with a gradual conditioning program.

Links to Experience

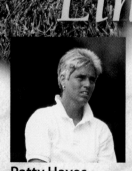

Patty Hayes

During the third round of the 1984 Samaritan Turquoise Classic in Arizona, Patti Hayes' iron shot to a green came up much too short. Frustrated and angry, she threw her club in the air and, to be sure the club got the message, tried to kick the shaft with her shoe. She missed, and hit her ankle against the club head instead. She kicked the club so hard she had to stop playing and wrap her foot in ice. She limped through the rest of the round and headed to the hospital for x-rays. Luckily, nothing was broken. "It was stupid. I learned a lesson. When you have a fight with a club, the club always wins."

Cramping in the calves of the leg while walking should not always be attributed to muscle strain. If, while walking, you experience pain in your calf that is relieved when you rest, this may be a reflection of a circulation problem called claudication. This vascular problem is the result of a blockage that interferes with the blood supply to the leg muscles. When you are walking down the fairway, those leg muscles need an adequate blood supply. If a blockage is present, blood supply will decrease and you will experience pain or aches in the calf that will be relieved when you rest. This problem frequently occurs in individuals who are smokers. If you find that after you hit your drive, you must stop one or two times before you reach your ball, you might want to consult your physician.

Remember, by keeping up with your walking, you will prevent further muscle soreness. The exercise will maintain your fitness, improve your tempo, and do great things for your cardiovascular system.

The Foot

Playing a round of golf requires more than 6500 steps. Five percent of golf injuries occur in the foot and ankle. In addition, many pre-existing foot and ankle problems can be aggravated by golf. Since the proper golf swing generally starts with more weight on the right side at address and impact, with a shift to the left side after contact and the follow-through, it's safe to assume that any injury or pain in either foot will impair swing mechanics.

A common injury due to chronic stress on the foot is plantar fasciitis. The plantar fascia is the tissue on the bottom surface of the foot and heel. It is under constant stress when we walk or run. When this tissue becomes inflamed, pain results upon every step. The pain can be nearly intractable, making it difficult to walk much less play golf. The treatment generally requires rest or perhaps the use of a splint at night. Splinting can alleviate pain and reduce inflammation. Plantar fasciitis can become a chronic condition aggravated by repeated injury. If you have this problem, use a cart for four to six weeks.

Bunions are extremely common. Generally they are caused by friction and pressure from footwear and aggravated by poorly fitted golf shoes. They are ten times more common in women, probably because of footwear. Treatment for bunions generally consists of changing to shoes that allow plenty of room between the forefoot and the inner lining of the shoe.

The "pump bump" is that occasional painful prominence on the back of the heel that results from the pressure of the shoe. Changing shoes or padding the heel will reduce the inflammation.

Corns are another common problem of the foot. A corn is the result of several layers of skin that occur over a bony prominence. It is the body's attempt to protect the skin over that prominence. As these layers increase, so does the pressure from socks and shoes, which results in pain. The treatment for corns requires reducing the pressure over the prominence. When not playing golf, consider switching to sandals or open-toe shoes.

Since golf is not always played on sunny days in the short grass, we may find ourselves stepping in mud or in casual water. Waterproofed and breathable golf shoes will protect our feet and maintain comfort. When your feet are wet the heat loss is twenty-three times faster than dry conductive loss. Furthermore, wet skin is susceptible to blisters and abrasion. When your feet perspire and moisture cannot escape, there may be swelling of your skin, your socks, and your shoes all together. This tight fit results in increasing pressure and subsequent injury to your skin.

Health Tip Purchase your shoes late in the day because feet tend to swell during the day.

Blisters are one of the most common injuries to the foot. They are the result of skin rubbing against another surface, causing friction and tearing the upper layers of the skin. Prevention requires minimizing the friction. Golf shoes should fit comfortably. Acrylic socks are less likely to retain moisture and cause friction than cotton socks. Drying agents, such as foot powder and spray antiperspirants, can reduce moisture. Blisters are treated to relieve pain and to avoid infection. A small blister requires no treatment. A large blister should be drained after it is cleaned with antibiotic

Links to Experience

Bernhard Langer, two-time U.S. Masters champion, feels a golf shoe "needs to be comfortable and provide stability for powerful leg action. The last thing I need is to have tired legs and feet when playing the final and deciding holes of a big tournament."

Bernhard Langer

soap, and then it should be covered with a dressing for ten to fourteen days.

Foot odor is caused by bacteria. To eliminate odor, scrub your feet with antibacterial soap and make sure your feet are dry (use a hair dryer). Wear absorbent socks and change them frequently.

Don't forget to watch out for the cart. Every year foot and ankle injuries occur due to carelessness (forgetting to secure the brake) and poor driving, including DWI. Senior Tour player Jim Albus was sidelined when a cart was backed into his leg. The injury required medical treatment and forced him to curtail his playing schedule.

TREATMENT AND PREVENTION OF FOOT INJURY: WHAT YOU SHOULD DO

- Plantar fasciitis requires modified activity, anti-inflammatory agents, stretching exercises, and possibly the use of a splint.
- Blisters and bunions can be avoided by choosing properly fitting shoes and wearing acrylic socks over cotton socks for less friction.
- Choose a golf shoe that is waterproof as well as breathable.
- Blisters, if large, should be cleaned, drained, and covered with antibiotic ointment and dressing.

Exercises for Plantar Fasciitis

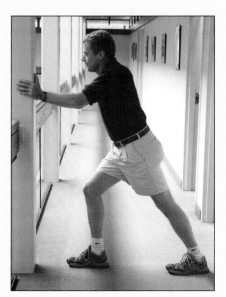

1. Plantar fasciitis stretch
Extend the affected foot back, and slowly push the heel of the affected foot toward the floor. Hold for 30 seconds, and repeat three times. Move the affected foot farther back as your flexibility improves.

Exercises for Plantar Fasciitis, continued

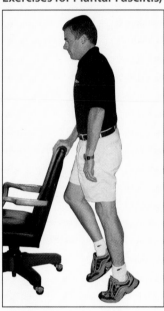

1. Plantar fasciitis stretch
Stand on the affected foot and rise up on toes. Slowly lower your heel back to the floor.

The Neck

Although neck pain represents only 5 percent of injuries to the golfer, it can be quite painful and disabling.

The problem may be in your cervical spine, but your symptoms are elsewhere—weakness or pain in your arm. If the pain is localized to your neck, it may be a muscle or ligament strain. Pain that radiates to the arms implies nerve involvement, possibly the result of a herniated disc with compression of the nerve root. If the discomfort increases with activity or a few hours after activity and settles down with rest, it probably is the result of mechanical irritation of the nerve. This is often due to a degenerative process or simply overuse. Relief comes with rest and anti-inflammatory agents.

Muscle spasms in the neck are overdiagnosed. Spasms can occur with acute injury, but their long-term presence indicates a deeper pain source.

TREATMENT AND PREVENTION OF NECK PAIN: WHAT YOU SHOULD KNOW

- Overuse is the culprit; rest is the cure.
- Use anti-inflammatory agents.
- When looking at a computer screen, keep it at eye level.
- Sleep on your side with arms at chest level.

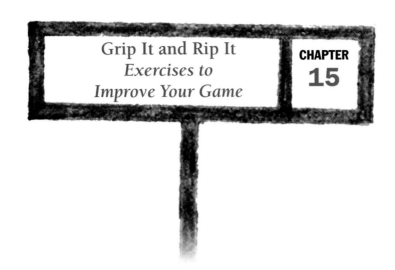

Grip It and Rip It
Exercises to
Improve Your Game

CHAPTER
15

Golfers find it a very trying matter to turn at the waist, more particularly if they have a lot of waist to turn.

—Harry Vardon

Golf needs to be considered exercise just like any other sport. It requires coordination, athletic movement, accuracy, strength, endurance, and flexibility. If there is any doubt that flexibility can contribute to the length of drives, observe the swing of John Daly (don't try this at home). Nearly every muscle in the body is involved in golf. Because of the demands on the body and the risk of injury, most professional golfers engage in structured exercise and flexibility programs. Unfortunately, bad backs are the most frequent injury on the tour and have affected many players including Lee Trevino, Jack Nicklaus, and Fred Couples. For everyone, from the professional to the weekend golfer, exercise and strength training are as important as practice on the putting green.

Professionals work at all aspects of their game to improve. After a round, if it is two or three beers then time to head home, it's not likely that the professional will make many cuts. A fitness trailer and a trainer, sponsored by Centinela Hospital and the PGA Tour, travel to all tournament stops. More and more professionals are using this facility and expertise; the benefits of exercise on athletic performance can't be overstated.

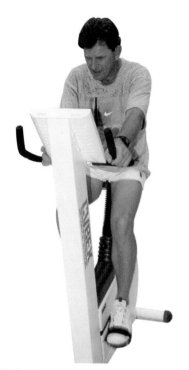

Nick Price

Centinela Hospital in Inglewood, California, established the research center where Tom Kite was evaluated. Now a strong advocate of golf-specific conditioning, he admits to having had little understanding of its importance early in his career. Lee Trevino, who suffered from a ruptured disk, estimates that fifty percent of tour players have back problems. He now incorporates back exercises into his practice regimen. Fitness awareness is not limited to the men's tour. Women on the LPGA Tour are no exception, seeking to improve their strength and cardiovascular endurance through training. Nancy Lopez routinely performs 200 abdominal crunches a day.

It is never too late to build strength. Studies have shown that sixty- and seventy-year-olds who exercise on a weight machine can increase their strength by 100 to 225 percent. For you, this increased strength could mean reaching the green in regulation or finally carrying that water hazard where you have donated so many balls.

Gary Player, three-time Masters champion, winner of the British Open in three different decades, and holder of 150 other tournament wins, attributes his success to fitness. For the past four years, Player has committed himself to fitness and strength training. At age sixty, he continues to participate in exercise that enhances his ability to play golf. He enjoys a reputation as one of the game's fittest golfers. It is not surprising, then, that Player is strongly opposed to the use of electric carts.

Strength Training and Muscular Endurance

We can lengthen the distance of our drives by increasing club-head speed. To accomplish this, golfers require strong muscle groups in the legs and forearms.

The forearms and wrists help to maintain a firm grip. The back muscles assist in swinging the arms through the swing plane.

Commitment to a specific strengthening and conditioning program will improve flexibility, prevent fatigue, and reduce the likelihood of injury. Contrary to opinion, muscle strengthening and weight lifting will not hurt your game. Exercises to increase strength involve use of resistance equipment, free weights, and calisthenics.

Myth: Weight lifting will hurt your golf game.
Truth: Golf-specific strengthening exercises can increase distance and reduce injury.

Endurance is an important element of your strengthening program. To build endurance when you exercise, do more repetitions and use less resistance. Endurance will enable you to avoid fatigue, whether it means you can play two days in a row or keep your concentration and focus on those final holes.

Your abdominal muscles help support your trunk and provide stability to your back. Abdominal crunches will help strengthen these areas. Forearm strength is necessary to maintain a good grip—check John Daly's "grip it and rip it" approach. Squeezing a rubber ball with fifty to seventy-five repetitions, or doing wrist curls, will imprOOve forearm strength. While walking eighteen holes requires leg strength, remember that the power for the drive is initiated in the lower body.

> *Winning at golf is total commitment, physically and mentally. If you feel you are weak, you should be in the gym developing your body for golf.*
>
> *Nick Faldo*

Curtis Strange found running on the course (not during play) a great way to condition his legs. If you have a bad back, consider cycling instead of running, because it involves much less trauma to the joints. When you begin a new exercise program, do as many repetitions as you can without pain. Increase the holding times and repetitions as you get more comfortable with the routines. And check with your physician before starting any exercise regime.

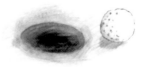

Strengthening Exercises

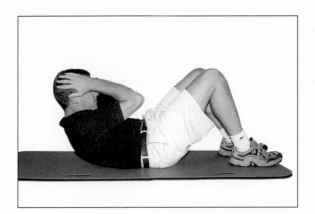

Abdominal crunches
10 to 30 reps
Hold hands by ears, keep chin tucked in, lift and hold, lower slowly.

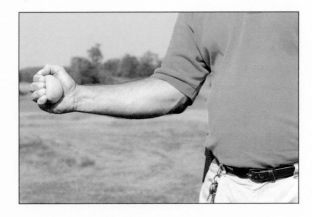

Ball squeeze
10 to 50 reps
Hold a rubber ball in each hand, squeeze rhythmically until the muscles are fatigued.

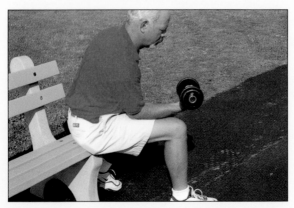

Wrist Curl
10 to 30 reps
Sit with wrists resting on knees, hold a bar or weight in each hand, twist up and down.

Golf can be a healthful activity. Walk the course and you can burn up to 470 calories per round—more if you carry your bag. The heart of the matter is this: to play good golf you need to be fit. If you play frequently and choose to walk, you can lower your cholesterol—and maybe your handicap.

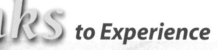

Links to Experience

Gary Player

"For nearly as long as I can remember, exercise has been part of my life. For many years I awoke before dawn, lifted weights at the Y and ran on the golf course—everybody thought I was nuts." Gary Player still works out for at least one hour, four times a week. Player, who was initially regarded as a short hitter, feels it was through exercise and training that he was able to increase his distance off the tee. Today in his sixties, Gary Player remains active and competitive on the Senior Tour and attributes his success and longevity in golf to exercise and proper training.

Stretching and Warm-Up

CHAPTER
16

Make up your mind before your backswing starts, then let your muscles do the work.

—Tommy Armour

Weekend golfers are slow starters and generally play the first few holes poorly. Lack of a warm-up may be to blame.

Drive balls at the course early. And stretch before swinging! Get those muscles ready to shoot that career round. With the proper warm-up, you increase the flow of blood and oxygen to your muscles and joints. A good stretching program is an effective way of preventing injury and avoiding those pulls and strains. To be effective, a proper program should include activity that elevates body temperature, such as a slow jog or a 5 to 10-minute walk. At the range, begin swinging the club slowly, and gradually increase the swing speed. Start with the heaviest club, the sand wedge, and make short swings. Gradually increase your arc with each club. Finish with your driver, then head to the tee. Muscles that are warm and stretched out prior to teeing off are supple and loose, enabling the body to perform to its full capability, and making it less likely to sustain injury.

Stretching and Warm-Up Exercises

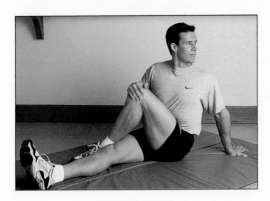

1. Hip stretch (sitting) Slowly pull your left knee toward your right side and hold to a count of 15. Stretch the right knee toward the left side.

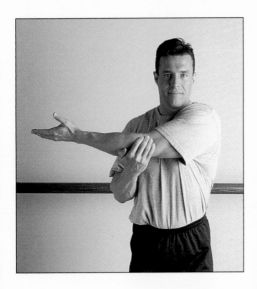

2. Shoulder stretch (left) Slowly pull your arm in toward your chest and hold to a count of 15. Stretch both shoulders.

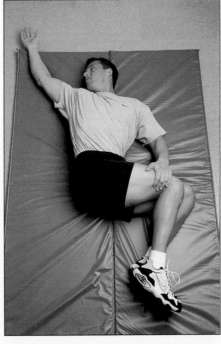

3. Trunk rotation (lying) (right) This a more advanced stretch than the back rotation exercise shown in Chapter 14. Lie on your side with your legs bent. Hold your thigh, reach over your head with your right arm, and slowly lower your shoulder as close to the floor as you can. Hold to a count of 15. Repeat from the opposite side.

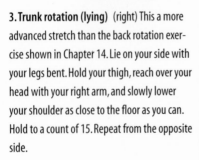

Stretching and Warm-Up Exercises, continued

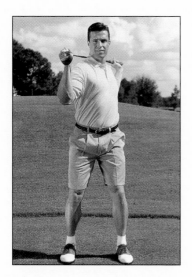

4. Trunk rotation (before the round) (left) Keep your knees bent slightly and your hips still. Slowly rotate your upper torso to one side and hold for a count of 5 seconds. Repeat on the other side.

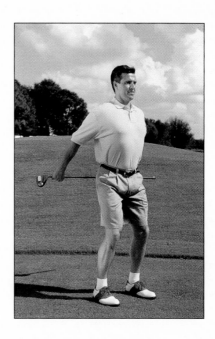

5. Chest stretch (before the round) (right) With your palms up, grasp a club behind you. Raise the club while pushing your chest outward, and breathe deeply. Hold to a count of 15. Don't forget to breathe.

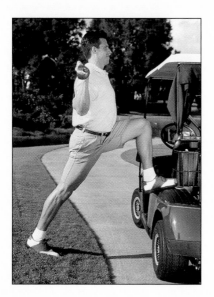

6. Hip and thigh stretch (during the round) (left) While keeping your forward knee directly over your ankle, slowly move your hips forward. Hold to a count of 15. Repeat with the other leg.

Stretching and Warm-Up Exercises, continued

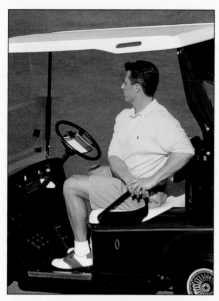

7. Trunk rotation (during the round)
(right) Keep your hips still and turn your body in one direction while looking over your shoulder in another. Hold to a count of 15.

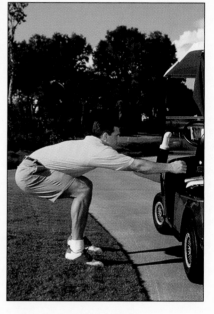

8. Lower back stretch (during the round) (left) Extend your arms and push your hips and buttocks backward. Hold to a count of 15. Don't forget to breathe.

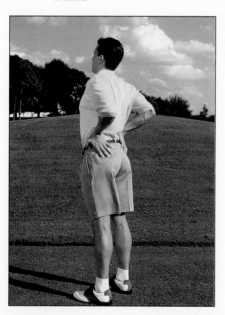

9. Back stretch (after the round)
(right) Place your hands on hips as shown. Arch your back slightly and tighten your stomach muscles. Hold to a count of 15. Don't forget to breathe.

Stretching and Warm-Up Exercises, continued

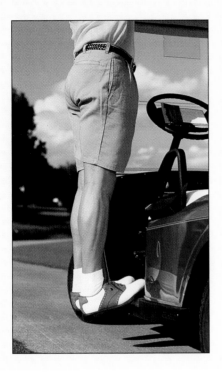

10. Calf stretch (after the round)
Lower your heels over the edge of a step
or cart. Hold to a count of 15.

Flexibility and the Senior Golfer

myth&TRUTHS

To play our best golf requires a combination of
strength, flexibility, and endurance. As we age, flexibility
and strength decrease, but both can be improved by swinging a weighted club. An exercise program can enhance and
maintain flexibility. Peter Egosue, who worked with Jack
Nicklaus, is a strong proponent of adequate flexibility. This
means allowing the muscles to work the way they were
designed. A few of the professionals who have adopted his
philosophy, and have extended their competitive careers,
include Sandra Palmer, Johnny Miller, and Dave Stockton.

Myth: Hitting a bucket
of balls before a round
loosens up your muscles
so you can avoid injury.
Truth: Swinging at a
bucket of balls is no substitute for adequate
warm-up and stretching
before going to the first
tee.

Flexibility exercises designed specifically for the back and
hips are helpful to maintain the distance of our drives and avoid
injury. Stretching is another way to promote flexibility. As with any exercise, listen to your body. If you have specific pains or feel tired after an
exercise session, cut back and take a rest.

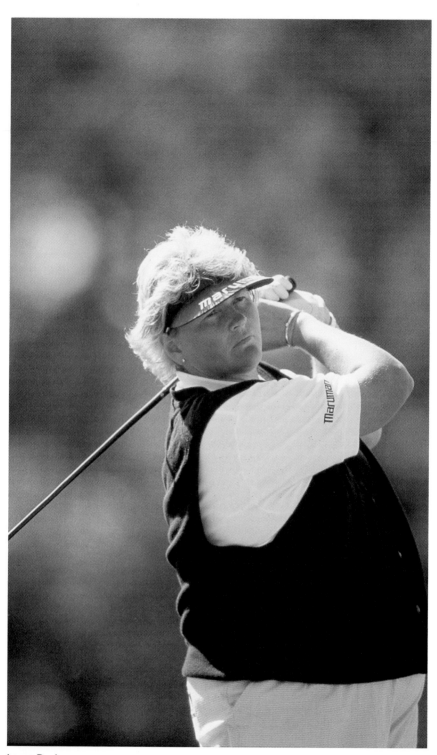

Laura Davies

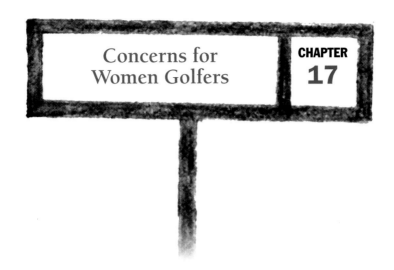

Concerns for
Women Golfers

CHAPTER
17

Laura Davies doesn't yell 'Fore,' she yells 'Liftoff.' You don't watch her ball, you track it, an unidentified flying object entering orbit.

—Jim Murray

Fitness

Optimum fitness for women should focus on cardiovascular conditioning, muscular endurance, muscular strength, and flexibility. Since women have only about two-thirds of the muscle mass of men, they often have more difficulty generating power. On the other hand, they do have a lower center of gravity, making balance much easier. The majority of amateur women players have difficulty maintaining a hold on their clubs because of weak wrist and forearm muscles. In fact, the most frequent injury on the women's professional tour is to the wrist.

To strengthen the hands and the arms, use a 3-lb weight in each hand and swing back and forth. You should build up repetitions and slowly increase the amount of weight over a period of months. Swinging a weighted club is another way of strengthening the wrist and forearms.

Wrist curls (see exercises 3 and 4 on page 125) are an excellent way to add strength to your hands and wrists.

Pregnant Golfers

Women can safely enjoy and participate in playing golf even while pregnant. Because your body is undergoing constant change, some adjustments need to be made to your game as well as to your swing. For example, Tammie Green, an LPGA Professional, had to contend with mild nausea in her first trimester, and during her last trimester, she needed antacids to alleviate her heartburn. She played her best golf during her second trimester. Because lower back pain frequently arises during pregnancy, strengthening the back muscles may help.

Another adaptation to her game was the need to stop five or six times during a round to use the facilities. This may present a greater problem for the average player, since portable facilities are not as available as they are in tournament play. Knowing this will be an issue, you will need to plan in advance. Fatigue associated with pregnancy, and concern over where the next restroom is located, may cause you to lose focus. Green found this not to be a problem since, as she remarked, "I only have to focus for one to two minutes over each shot."—A good lesson for all of us.

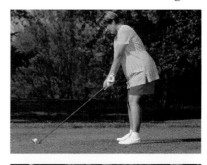

Blood vessels tend to dilate during pregnancy and may lower a woman's blood pressure. Keeping yourself hydrated by drinking plenty of water while playing will minimize the dizziness often associated with lower blood pressure. Extreme high blood pressure during pregnancy, on the other hand, is a potentially dangerous complication. If this is a problem for you, you should check with your obstetrician before playing. Pregnancy alters your body with both breast and abdominal enlargement. Tammy Green found that cutting her putter down one inch enabled her to avoid interference from her abdomen. Holding the hands a bit higher and flattening the swing plane also will allow you to maintain good mechanics.

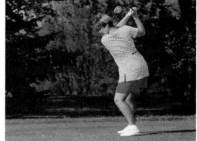

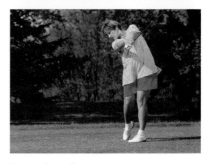

You can play your best golf while pregnant. Knowing what to expect and making adjustments to the natural changes in your body will help your game.

Nancy Ramsbottom

THE PREGNANT GOLFER: WHAT YOU SHOULD KNOW

- ■ Anticipate the need for frequent urination.
- ■ Because adequate hydration is essential, drink plenty of water and avoid diuretics.
- ■ Take calcium-based antacids (like Tums) to manage heartburn.
- ■ Try making adjustments in your swing plane and shortening the length of your putter by an inch.

Menopause and Golf

Menopause is associated with hormonal changes, diminished strength, and endurance. Exercise through golf can prevent or minimize many of the problems associated with menopause.

Today we know that exercise, including walking, can reduce night sweats and hot flashes. Loss of muscle mass also occurs at this time and can clearly affect your ability to maintain endurance and drive for distance. Strength training, as part of your overall golf fitness program, can substantially increase your muscle strength. Although women have minimal testosterone, they can develop strength without having large muscles.

Women at this time of their lives are at risk for bone loss due to osteoporosis. It is estimated that by the age of sixty, a woman easily can lose fifteen to thirty percent of her peak bone mass. Osteoporosis is the loss of bone mass, and it results in thinning bones that are susceptible to fractures. Estrogen, either naturally produced by the body or in the form of supplements, assists bone growth by helping calcium get absorbed by the body.

The best way to prevent osteoporosis is a combination of estrogen replacement, adequate calcium intake (dairy products are best), and exercise. Since walking is a great exercise to maintain bone density and ward off the complications of weak bones, why not do it on the course?

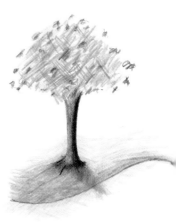

Strengthening Exercises for Women Golfers

When you begin a new exercise program, do as many repetitions as you can without pain. Increase the holding times and repetitions as you get more comfortable with the routines. And check with your physician before starting any exercise regime.

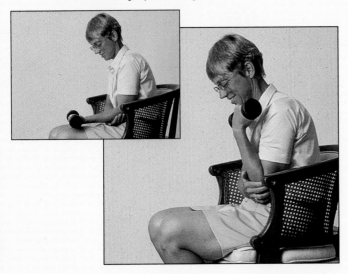

1. Biceps Rest your arm on your lap, palm up (inset). Support the arm with your other hand placed just below the elbow. Raise the handweight slowly to shoulder level (large photo), then lower at the same rate.

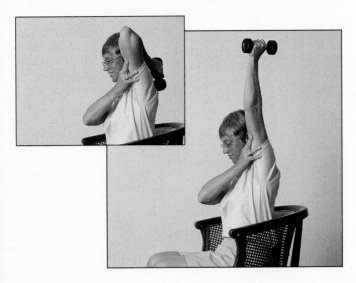

2. Triceps Bend your arm and raise your elbow so it is pointing straight up (inset). Support your uplifted arm with your other hand and straighten your arm slowly without altering the position of the elbow (large photo).

Strengthening Exercises for Women Golfers, continued

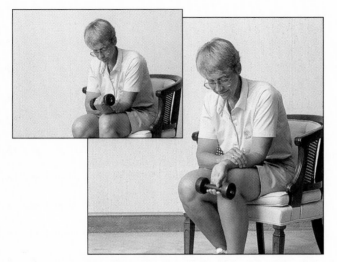

3. Anterior of forearm With weight in hand and your palm facing up, rest one arm on your leg with your wrist extended on your knee (inset). Support your forearm with your other hand. Let the handweight roll onto your fingers slowly (large photo), then curl your hand upward as far as possible so the weight rolls back into your palm.

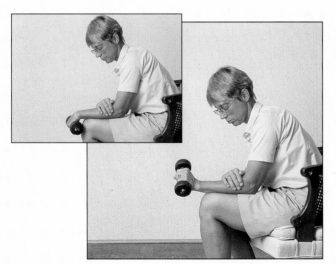

4. Posterior of forearm Assume the same starting position as in Exercise 3, except your palm faces down instead of up (inset). Let the handweight pull your knuckles toward the floor, then curl them upward slowly as far as you can (large photo).

Strengthening Exercises for Women Golfers, continued

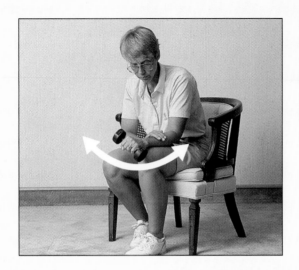

5. Rotator muscles of the wrist and the elbow Assume the same starting position as in Exercise 3. Rotate the weight slowly as far as you can, and then back in the opposite direction as shown by the arrow.

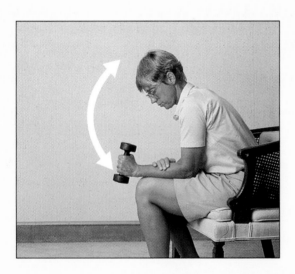

6. Another wrist strengthener Again from the same starting position, but with the back of your hand facing to your left as shown, hold the handweight firmly and raise your hand so your thumb moves toward your body. Now lower your hand slowly.

Strengthening Exercises for Women Golfers, continued

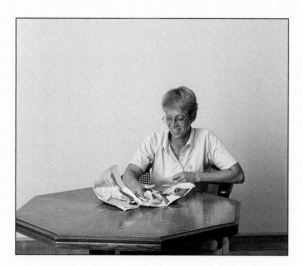

7. Hands An easy way to increase strength and suppleness in your hands and fingers is to crumple some old newspapers. Simple place a page on a table and, keeping your palm face down, crumple it into as small a ball as possible.

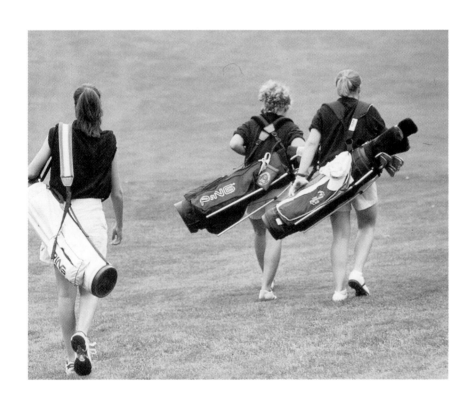

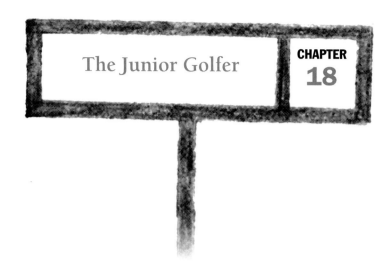

The Junior Golfer

CHAPTER 18

*Golf, like measles, should be caught young, or, if it is
postponed to ripe years, the results may be serious.*

—P. G. Wodehouse

You don't have to start playing golf at age five to be good. Many accomplished players, like Ernie Els, started to play in early adolescence and have developed into great players. Hiromi Kobayashi began at age eighteen. Young golfers have the opportunity to participate in various junior programs sponsored by local clubs and regional or national golfing organizations. The young men and women who play competitive golf may be prone to the problems of stress and anxiety as well as overuse injuries from repetitive practice.

The girl who competes in high school often must make the "boys' team." My daughter, Marliese, played in this situation for her four years in high school and always was required to play from the men's tee. However, a girl on the "boys' team" often has the psychological advantage of always having the boys attempt to outdrive her—but overswinging rarely results in a well-executed shot.

Today, thanks to Title IX legislation for equality, the opportunity for more women's teams in collegiate golf is greater.

Adolescence

The biological, social, and emotional changes that occur during adolescence can affect your ability to play golf. As you progress through adolescence, you will increase your strength and improve your motor skills performance. At some point in your adolescence, you will experience a rapid gain in height and weight. Your change in height has a dramatic effect on the equipment you use (length of shaft and swing) as well as your swing plane.

Swings in emotion are normal during your adolescence. You will need to work on keeping them under control, especially in competitive situations. Junior players, I have observed, are more likely to become exasperated after a poor shot. I've seen cases in which young players throw their clubs down in disgust or exhibit facial expressions of disbelief when their putts didn't drop. (You'd think that, after observing these facial responses and body actions, somehow the laws of nature and gravity had been violated.) I remember an excellent junior player who, after hitting a poor tee shot, hit the signpost with his fist. He was sidelined for the remainder of the season with a fractured hand. Keep in mind that the golfers who make the college teams haven't just demonstrated a high level of proficiency. They've developed a proper program of conditioning, good habits, and a positive mental attitude that has enabled them to compete at this level. Nevertheless, junior and collegiate players are not immune from problems of stress that range from alcohol addiction to asthma attacks. John Daly's struggle with alcohol began in adolescence. Hank Kuehne overcame similar problems and went on to win the recent U.S. Amateur competition.

Juniors and Fitness

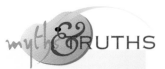

Myth: Women who do strength training develop large muscles.

Truth: Strengthening the muscles does not mean they will become enlarged.

Fitness is just as important in the junior golfer as it is in the older player. Adolescents can adjust to a training program and improve fitness much more quickly than older players. Today's collegiate standouts like Grace Park and Jimmy Chausiriporn eat nutritious foods, run, stretch, and pump iron. Park routinely hits the ball 250 yards. Strength training for girls and boys can be helpful to improve the length of their drives and avoid fatigue.

The Strength Training Controversy

Controversy has surrounded strength training in young people because of the possibility of damage to the growth plate in skeletally immature youth. Most injuries to the growth plate are from trauma or are the result of poor technique — trying to lift too much weight. Recent studies with bone scans show no damage to bone or muscle as a result of strength training programs.

Adolescents, as well as the adults, need to adhere to a regimen that includes no more than three strength sessions per week with a proper warm-up, a stretching session, and a cool-down. They should begin their programs without weights so they can practice good techniques and control.

Juniors' Injuries and Illnesses

Despite your enviable flexibility and resilience, you are not exempt from injury and are subject to problems of overuse. Repetitive practice may result in injuries to the back and elbow. It's typical at this age to want to hit for distance — it's hard to contain your energy. Suddenly you've acquired so much strength that you may want to swing as hard as you can. A junior player may be highly competitive and attempt to swing harder to outdrive his or her competitors, be it on the range or first tee. You run the risk of injury if you overswing to impress friends or peers. The need for girls to keep pace and play at the same level of the boys in order to secure a position on the team also raises issues of possible injury.

Most junior players believe themselves to be physically invincible and do not accept the reality of illness. You need to realize that if you have a viral or flu-like illness, rest is required and you can't return immediately to playing golf.

Because of your age, you may be prone to asthma. The asthma is brought on by the multiple allergens on the course from pollens, dust, molds, and pesticides. It can vary from a mild cough and wheeze to severe shortness of breath and difficulty breathing.

The psychological stress of tournament play may be especially difficult for the younger player. If not monitored properly, stress can precipitate an asthma attack. Even vigorous exercise can initiate an attack. If you have a history of asthma, you need to be aware of the signs of an impending attack and to take your medication and inhalers appropriately and in time. Anticipate an attack. Knowing when to take the medication and its possible side effects (such as feeling hyper or experiencing a tremor) are essential. They can affect not only your putting, but your health as well.

Links to Experience

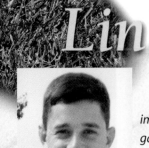

Mike Drepanos

—By Mike Depranos

Learning the game of golf is a long process, and it is important to remember that, beyond all else, it is just a game. As children start getting better at the game, they become interested in playing tournaments to test their skills. At a young age it is pure fun. No one really cares who comes in first or last. Somewhere along the way, however, children lose sight of the real reason they became interested in the game and put too much pressure on themselves. Goals become necessity rather than natural occurrences. If a junior breaks 80, then he or she is expected to do it every time.

I noticed that, when growing up, some pressure to do well in golf comes from within. This is very manageable and even a driving force to enjoy the game more. Pressure to do well becomes a problem when outside forces interfere, such as parents. I have seen talented young players burn out because their parents pushed them too hard. Some parents insist that their children practice and make them take lessons to improve. Overenthusiastic parents force their children to play in tournaments and yell at them for making poor shots or not placing well. These are the types of parents who typically watch their son or daughter hit every shot at the range and constantly critique them.

Growing up playing the game, I've experienced all types of players. I've seen players with tremendous abilities fall short of being spectacular. I've also seen kids with less talent become very successful because of their mental abilities. Learning how to swing and make good shots is only one aspect of the game. The other side is mental — in my opinion the more important side of golf. You have to be mentally tough to play this game well.

Golf is about overcoming and regathering yourself. One talented friend of mine did not perform well in tournaments because he had so much pressure on him. The first poor shot he hit usually resulted in a temper tantrum. He would often curse or throw clubs. Once he gave in to his temper, his game would go up in flames. He would self-destruct. I watched him do it time and time again. In one extreme circumstance, I saw him punch a post after hitting a meager shot. Not only did that ruin his round, but it also ruined his summer. After the round, he found out he broke his hand and he was sidelined for the entire summer and fall.

Another friend of mine was a tremendous success growing up. He was so used to winning that he really did not know what it was like to lose. But one bad hole had an effect not only on his golf game, but on his life. He was in the third round of an American Junior Golf Association tournament and was winning by four shots with three holes to play. He had a large gallery and TV cameras following him. The tournament was seemingly in the bag. However, he hit multiple balls out of bounds on his way to a thirteen. He went on to lose the tournament and his self-esteem. He never recovered from this tournament.

I have learned from these players' mistakes. I realize that the game can go from being the most satisfying game to the most depressing game. That is why I like to take the game for what it is. I have had my share of up times and down times, but I always try to keep my head up. One summer in an AJGA tournament held at my home course, I shot a 94 in the final round and followed it up the very next summer by shooting a 70. It is important to remember to block out the bad rounds and focus on the good rounds. Always remember that it is just a game.

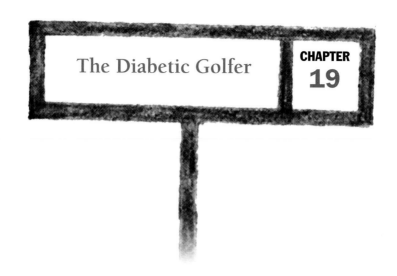

The Diabetic Golfer

CHAPTER 19

Nothing is impossible to a willing heart.

—John Heywood

Diabetes is certainly not a reason to avoid golf. Michelle McGann, at age nineteen, was one of the youngest woman to join the LPGA Tour. Diagnosed with the condition at age thirteen, she followed a variety of regimens to control her disease, including taking insulin. Michelle, like many diabetics, monitors her glucose and takes insulin. She also plays excellent golf.

Sherri Turner, the 1988 LPGA money winner, and Kellie Kuehne are diabetic. Scott Verplank, who competes on the men's tour, is also able to deal effectively with this disease.

Diabetes is a common medical condition. Even so, not long ago the terms "diabetic" and "athlete" seemed to be mutually exclusive. Today, most physicians encourage diabetic patients to exercise. Exercise is important to everyone's health, but it's especially important to diabetics. A Pittsburgh study found that the number of complications that arise from diabetes can be reduced by playing sports.[5]

Medication

Diabetics who are dependent on insulin may find that regular exercise through playing golf can in fact reduce the amount of insulin the body requires. Physical training can also help prevent the resistance to insulin that occurs as

134

the result of obesity. If you are an avid golfer, play frequently, and walk the course, consider reducing your insulin dosage by ten percent. Reduction of the insulin dose should be based on regular blood sugar checks on golfing days. The exact amount of insulin to reduce should be discussed with your physician. For those of you who control your blood sugar with pills, playing golf on a regular basis may enable you to reduce the dosage of this medication as well. Exercise can improve the control of the blood sugar and reduce fat storage for people who have diabetes and are not on insulin.

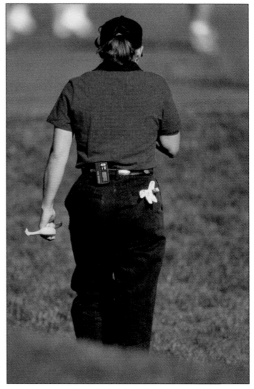

Kellie Kuehne wears a blood sugar monitor on her belt.

Any exercise, including golf, can influence the rate at which insulin is absorbed from the injection site into the blood. Golfers should not inject insulin into their arms within an hour of playing. The muscle activity of swinging the club will force the insulin into the bloodstream faster than usual, resulting in low blood sugar. If you walk the course, avoid injections to the leg muscles for the same reason. The abdomen is the best spot for injection of insulin on a golfing day.

If the blood sugar is under good control, you should consider increasing your food intake prior to playing because your blood sugar may decrease while golfing. Foods rich in carbohydrates, such as bread, crackers, and pasta are the best choices. The amount of food you should eat depends on the pre-exercise blood sugar test. The most important nutrient one needs during exercise is water. Playing golf on a warm, humid day can result in the loss of large amounts of fluid. Thirst is generally not a good indication of how much fluid to drink.

When Not to Play

The diabetic golfer on insulin or large doses of diabetes pills should watch for symptoms of insulin reaction. Symptoms include extreme fatigue, sweatiness, shakiness, rapid heartbeat, dizziness, poor concentration, and even decreased performance at golf. If you are uncertain whether you are having a reaction, you should stop your golfing activity immediately. Don't finish the hole. Test your blood sugar if possible to confirm your symptoms.

If your blood sugar is low, take a sugar-containing food immediately. It is best that this food be in the form of a simple sugar (hard candy, juice, regular soda) rather than a more complex form, such as a candy bar or cookie. Now rest in order to allow the body to equilibrate and absorb the glucose. If the next scheduled meal or snack is more than a half hour away, eat a slow-acting carbohydrate and a source of protein. Crackers with peanut butter are a good choice . You can then return to the links and finish your round.

In the case of an insulin-dependent diabetic whose blood sugar is greater than 300 and spilling ketones in the urine, it is best not to golf on that day. In this situation, exercise does not decrease the blood sugar. It actually sends it higher. Golf should also be avoided if your blood sugar is low, less than 60. Consult a physician immediately for advice about insulin adjustment.

Health Tip

The weather can upset the insulin-carbohydrate balance. Cold weather may slow the absorption of insulin, while hot weather may actually increase it.

Learning to Adjust

Lee Elder, Senior Tour player, has diabetes. This past March he noticed the sudden onset of double vision. After visiting his physician, he found out that he has nerve damage to his eye that may be permanent. He has elected to continue to play on the Tour despite the fact he must wear a patch over his left eye. With vision in only one eye he has no depth perception and is unable to tell how far to hit it or how to read a break.

The diabetic patient who is new to golf and exercise must learn how to adjust his or her diet and insulin dosage to accommodate the body's increased energy needs. The process is achieved best with frequent blood glucose monitoring, especially before and after a round. As with any medication, individualized care is extremely important. Adjustments that may work well for one individual may not apply to another. Learn how your body responds to the physical and emotional stresses of golf, as well as to competition, in order to regulate your diet and medication to achieve your full potential.

The diabetic golfer should also pay close attention to foot care. Fungal infections, abrasions, and blisters can become serious for the diabetic. Clean socks and correctly sized golf shoes are essential to avoid foot injuries.

Many individuals with diabetes have excelled in golf. But like all aspects of training in any sport, diabetic management requires discipline. Time and motivation are required to coordinate diet, exercise, and insulin injections.

Links to Experience

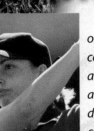

Kellie Kuehne

Kellie Kuehne, a former U.S. Amateur champion and 1999 winner of the LPGA Corning Classic, contends with not only making putts and playing against the toughest competition in the world, but also managing her diabetes. Kellie is an insulin dependent diabetic. Whether it's practice or playing competitively, she closely monitors her blood sugar. She even wears a device that constantly monitors her blood sugar during play and provides a warning beep if her sugar drops too low. She has been in situations in competitive play when her sugar dropped, causing her to lose focus and concentration.

Kellie remarked, "I always believed in me, and that's what got me to where I am. What are the odds? I'm five foot-two and I'm a diabetic. People would say, 'How could she make it?' But I've gotten here and believing in myself is a big part of it." She feels that having this problem has also been a blessing: "Having diabetes has made me more disciplined not only in golf, but in life."

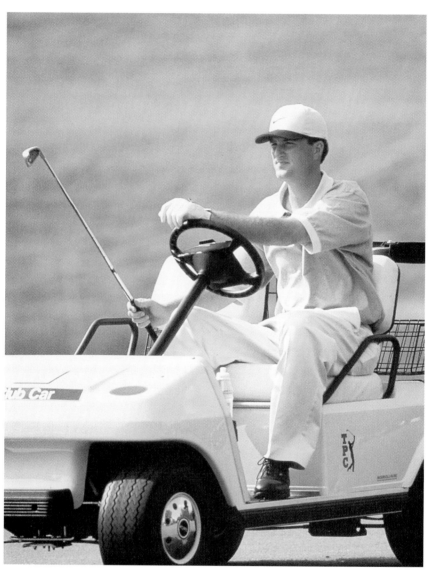

Casey Martin

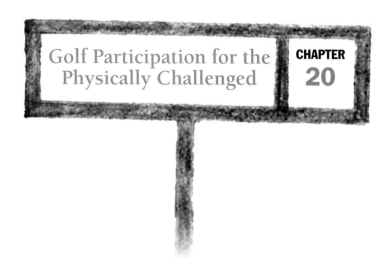

Golf Participation for the Physically Challenged

CHAPTER

20

Success in golf depends less on strength of the body than strength of the mind and character.

— Arnold Palmer

The nature of golf lends itself to participation by individuals of all abilities, including those who are physically challenged. Physically handicapped people out on the golf course range from those with artificial joints to amputees.

If you are a newly disabled golfer, you can use the game as part of your psychological and physical rehabilitation. Golf allows you to be competitive even with a nondisabled golfer. Through golf, you can develop skills of emotion, goal-setting, positive thinking, and acceptance of human limitations. With adjustments in equipment and technique, golf can be enjoyed by individuals with most disabilities.

Using prostheses, both lower and upper amputees can adjust to the game. Wheelchairs and even special golf carts from which to play have been designed. Visually impaired golfers can compete in tournaments run by the U.S. Blind Golfers Association. The golfers use coaches who line up shots and provide information on distance and direction.

Advances in medical technology have permitted many previously excluded individuals to enjoy the game. In addition to artificial prostheses, total joint replacement has assisted some players with severe arthritis. Julius Boros, former Senior Tour player, underwent total hip replacement while playing on the tour. Jack Nicklaus is now back on the Senior Tour after an artificial joint was placed in his left hip. For him, the option for surgery was a "quality of life issue."

For golfers who are physically challenged, there are individuals and organizations to assist and encourage them in the game of golf and help them reach their full potential. The Physically Challenged Golf Association and the National Amputee Golf Association have supported individuals with disabilities by creating awareness, and providing them with instruction and alternative equipment. The Professional Golf Association of America has established a committee for the physically challenged to develop instructional strategies and training guidelines for PGA professionals. The Hurdzien Design Group has even developed a nine-hole course for the handicapped player. In conjunction with the Edwin Shaw Rehabilitation Hospital in Akron, Ohio, the golf course was designed so that amputees and other players dependent on the use of wheelchairs and crutches can enjoy playing the game of golf rather than watching from the sidelines. The wheelchairs use wider wheels and greens are accessible through ramps. Bunkers have gentle slopes and tees are wider, making them easier to get on and off.

The Golf Writers Association of America annually gives the Ben Hogan Award to an individual who has continued to be active in golf despite a physical handicap. In 1949 Ben Hogan, the best player in the world, was involved in an automobile accident in which he was nearly killed. Having fractured twenty bones, he was not expected to live. His only wish was to be able to walk again. Not only did he achieve this goal but he was able to return to golf and go on to win the Masters, the U.S. Open, and the British Open in the same year! The 1999 recipient of the Ben Hogan award was Casey Martin.

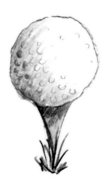

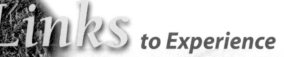

Links to Experience

Keith Harris is not your average amateur player to qualify for the Mid-Amateur. While in high school, he was run over by a car driven by his best friend and dragged 180 feet. His injuries included one ear ripped off, two broken arms, seven pints of blood lost, and virtually no skin left anywhere on his body. There was a large gaping hole in his back and both sacroiliac joints were dislocated. He was not expected to survive, but he did, and ultimately underwent twenty-two operations.

Six months after his accident, he played nine holes and shot forty-three. He said, "It hurt like hell, but I could do it and that was the important thing." His health problems continue with arthritis and tendonitis. During his convalescence he couldn't swing a club, "but," he said, "I've learned to chip and putt." He qualified for the Mid-Amateur and carries a handicap of a plus 1.6. "My view of life has changed 180 degrees. These years are bonus years. No one enjoys playing golf more than I do. I don't get upset about a bad shot any more."

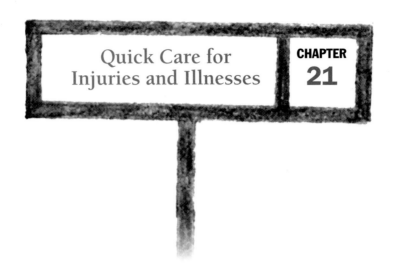

Quick Care for Injuries and Illnesses

CHAPTER 21

If your opponent is playing several shots in vain attempts to extricate himself from a bunker, do not stand near him and audibly count his strokes. It would be justifiable homicide if he wound up his pitiable exhibition by applying a niblick to your head.

— Henry Vardon

Most golfers, professional and recreational, suffer a golf-related injury sometime during their pursuit of the sport. The trauma from being hit by a ball or club can be very serious. Other possible injuries on the course include breaking a bone, spraining an ankle, or dislocating a joint after tripping over a rake or slipping on wet grass, being struck by lightning, getting run over by an electric cart, and even getting stung by a swarm of bees. Eyes can become injured by a blow from a club, a flying divot, or sand from a bunker. Recently, a thirty-five-year-old man from Naples, Florida, fell out of a cart, hit his head, and died as a result of the head injury.

The probability of being struck by a golf ball seemed relatively remote until the press highlighted the golfing exploits of former President Gerald Ford. Unfortunately, serious head injuries occur. A death resulting from an errant golf ball was reported as far back as the late 1800s. According to *Golf Digest*, nearly 40,000 golfers are admitted to emergency rooms each year after being hit with misdirected shots or flying club heads.[6] A study from Scotland reported that forty percent of sports-related head injuries in children were related to golf. Playing on crowded public courses increases the chance of being hit by an errant ball, especially if the parallel fairways are going in opposite directions.

Because accidents on the course can happen, it is important for all golfers to be able to recognize injuries and provide basic care to fellow golfers during the game.

Is the Golfer Injured?

When a golfer has been injured during play, your first actions are to find out:

- what happened
- how serious is the injury
- is the golfer conscious and breathing
- how did the injury occur

Call for Help When...

The golfer needs help when he or she is experiencing or has experienced:

- an altered mental status such as dizziness, confusion, or loss of consciousness
- breathing difficulty
- a cardiac arrest or apparent heart problems
- choking
- a diabetic emergency
- electrocution
- an inability to move or bear weight on a limb
- persistent or severe chest pain or discomfort
- a seizure
- a severe allergic reaction
- severe bleeding
- a severe headache
- severe weakness

Call or direct another golfer or golf staff member to call 911 or the local emergency number right away when a golfer has any of the listed problems. The person who answers the call will be an Emergency Medical Service (EMS) dispatcher, and this person will ask:

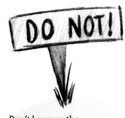

Don't hang up the telephone until the EMS dispatcher hangs up!

- your name
- the phone number from which you are calling
- the exact location of the emergency
- the nature of the emergency
- what happened
- the number of golfers who are ill or injured

Speak clearly; once the dispatcher knows what has happened, he or she will be able to tell you how to provide care until the ambulance arrives.

Allergic Reactions

Anaphylactic shock is a life-threatening allergic reaction in which the person may become unable to breathe and lose consciousness. Immediate intervention is necessary to save the ill golfer's life. If he or she has a history of bad allergic reactions to things like insect bites or stings, or even certain food, quickly call 911 or your local emergency number.

Signs to look for in a golfer having an allergic reaction are flushed and warm skin, hives, swelling, coughing or clearing of throat, difficulty breathing, cramps, and diarrhea.

Animal Bites

Any animal bite poses the risk of infection. Rabies in dogs has been virtually eliminated; today ninety-seven percent of reported rabies cases come from racoons, bats, skunks, and foxes.

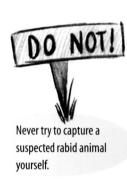

Never try to capture a suspected rabid animal yourself.

To care for a golfer with an animal bite:

1. Use direct pressure to control bleeding.
2. If bleeding is minor, wash the bite wound thoroughly with soap and water.

Signs of a rabid animal:

- The animal is unprovoked, yet attacks.
- The animal appears unusually hyperactive or vicious.
- The animal is a member of a high-risk species such as a bat, raccoon, skunk, or fox.

Bee and Insect Stings

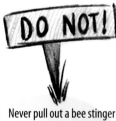

Never pull out a bee stinger with a venom sac still attached to it, with tweezers or your fingers; you may squeeze poisonous venom into the golfer!

To care for a conscious golfer with a bee sting:

1. See if a stinger is embedded in the golfer's skin, and check to see if it has a venom sac attached.
2. If you find a stinger, scrape it out with a fingernail or credit card.
3. Wash the area that has been stung with soap and water.
4. Apply an ice pack or cold compress for 15 to 20 minutes—even a cold soda can or bottle can help.
5. Observe the golfer for 30 minutes for signs of an allergic reaction.

6. If the golfer's breathing is affected:
   - Ask if he or she has a physician-prescribed epinephrine auto-injector, and if so, assist him or her in using it. It may be located in his or her golf bag.
   - Call 911 or your local emergency phone number immediately. The golfer may be in a life-threatening situation!
7. Cover the bite with a sterile dressing or clean cloth.

Bleeding

External bleeding is easy to recognize, but internal bleeding is slightly harder to detect. Signs to look for in a person who is bleeding internally are bruises on the skin — with or without pain — swelling of the skin, or the coughing up of blood.

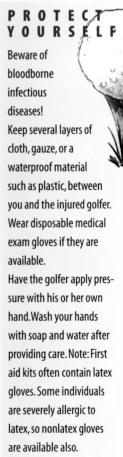

PROTECT YOURSELF

Beware of bloodborne infectious diseases! Keep several layers of cloth, gauze, or a waterproof material such as plastic, between you and the injured golfer. Wear disposable medical exam gloves if they are available. Have the golfer apply pressure with his or her own hand. Wash your hands with soap and water after providing care. Note: First aid kits often contain latex gloves. Some individuals are severely allergic to latex, so nonlatex gloves are available also.

To care for a golfer with minor external bleeding:
1. Wash the wound with soap and water, if available.
2. Cover the wound with a clean dressing; use your towel.
3. Apply pressure to the wound for a few minutes to stop the bleeding.
4. Apply an antibiotic ointment to the wounded area.
5. Cover the wound with an adhesive bandage, such as a Band-Aid®.

To care for a golfer with serious external bleeding:
1. Seek medical assistance.
2. Cover the wound with a clean dressing; use your towel.
3. Apply pressure to the wound for a few minutes to control the bleeding.
4. Elevate the injured area, if possible.
5. Maintain pressure on the wound by applying a gauze dressing and bandage.
6. If blood soaks through the bandage, do not remove it; apply another over the first.

To care for a golfer with internal bleeding, such as a bruise from a golf ball:

1. Limit movement of the injured area.
2. Apply ice.
3. Elevate the injured area, if possible.

Blisters

Signs to look for in a golfer with blisters are a raised bubble of skin covering clear liquid, or a broken flat piece of skin.

To care for a golfer with an unbroken blister that is mildly painful:

1. Cut doughnut-shaped holes in several gauze pads, moleskin, or molefoam to fit around the blister.
2. Tape the doughnut-shaped pads into place.

To care for a golfer with a broken blister:

1. Clean the area with soap and water.
2. Apply antibiotic ointment.
3. Apply doughnut-shaped pads around the blister and then cover it with an uncut gauze pad.

To care for a golfer with a blister that is painful and affects his or her ability to walk or participate:

1. Drain the fluid from the blister by making several small holes in it with a sterilized needle.
2. Clean the area with soap and water.
3. Apply antibiotic ointment.
4. Apply doughnut-shaped pads around the blister and then cover it with an uncut gauze pad.

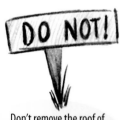

Don't remove the roof of the blister unless it is torn or painful and affects walking or participation.

Bone, Joint, and Muscle Injuries

Bone, joint, and muscle injuries are rarely life-threatening. Often, the best thing you can do is to help reduce the injured golfer's anxiety, and keep him or her from moving the injured area. Bone, joint, and muscle injuries share similar signs and symptoms, so it can often be difficult or impossible for you to determine the extent of the injury. Because of this, bone, joint, and muscle injuries are handled using similar techniques.

Signs to look for in a person who has a bone, joint, or muscle injury are deformity or angulation of a body part, pain and tenderness, crepitus (bone ends grating), swelling, bruising (discoloration), and exposed bone ends (open injury).

To care for a golfer with a bone, joint, or muscle injury:

1. Expose the affected area and look for bruising, swelling, deformity, or protruding bone ends.
2. Immobilize the injured area with a splint. You do not need a commercial splint to stabilize the injured area; you can use items such as your club, a rolled towel, a board, a magazine, or an uninjured body part.
3. Do not attempt to move the affected area, but splint it in the position you find it. Always place the splint so that the joints above and below the injury site cannot move. For example, if a golfer has a forearm injury, position the splint to extend beyond both his elbow and his wrist.
4. The splint should be long enough and wide enough to stabilize the injury.
5. If the golfer cannot move a limb, or has inured his or her head or neck, have him or her stay still, and call 911 or your local emergency number.
6. With the exception of open bone injuries, place a bag of ice over the affected area, elevate the splinted site, and compress the area using your golf towel.
7. Basic **RICE** guidelines for bone, joint, and muscle injuries:
   Rest - Do not move injured part.
   Ice - Apply ice for twenty-minute intervals.
   Compression - Compress the injured area with an elastic bandage during ice pack intervals.
   Elevation - Elevate the injured part above the heart.

Breathing Problems

Signs to look for in a golfer who is having a problem breathing are coughing, skin that looks more blue than pink, inability to complete sentences with one breath, and high-pitched sounds during breathing.

To care for a conscious golfer who is having problems breathing:

1. Have the golfer sit upright.
2. If the golfer has a physician-prescribed, hand-held inhaler, have him or her
   - exhale deeply,
   - place lips around the inhaler's opening,
   - depress the inhaler while inhaling, and
   - hold his or her breath for several seconds.
3. Call 911 or your local emergency number if the condition cannot be resolved.

To care for a golfer who is breathing very fast or deeply (hyperventilating):

1. Talk to the golfer in a reassuring and calm voice.
2. Encourage the golfer to take long, slow breaths, and to hold each breath before slowly exhaling.
3. Call 911 or your local emergency number if the golfer has a severe or prolonged episode.

To care for a golfer who is not breathing:

1. See if the golfer is conscious and responsive by tapping him or her on the shoulder and loudly asking, "Are you OK?"

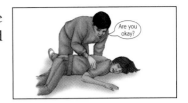

2. If the golfer does not respond, call or direct someone else to call 911 or your local emergency number immediately.

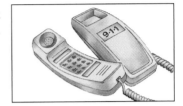

3. Gently roll the golfer onto his or her back.

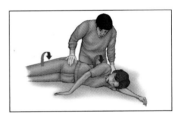

4. Tilt the golfer's head back and lift the chin. If you suspect a spinal injury, lift the chin but do not tilt the head back. Check for breathing by looking at the rise and fall of the chest, listening for breath sounds, and feeling for breaths on your cheek.

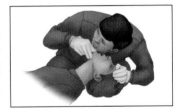

5. If the golfer is not breathing, give 2 slow breaths. If the first breath does not go in, retilt the head and give a second breath; if breaths still do not go in, the airway is probably blocked. (See Choking.)

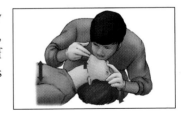

6. Check for a pulse in the neck. If a pulse is present, but the golfer still is not breathing, breath for him or her. Give 1 breath every 5 seconds.

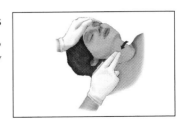

Choking

Signs to look for in a person who is conscious and choking are clasping of hands around throat (the universal distress signal) and the inability to make any sound.

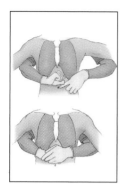

In the Conscious State

To care for a conscious golfer who is choking:

1. Ask the golfer, "Are you choking?" Someone who is choking will not be able to breathe, talk, cry, or cough.
2. Position yourself behind the golfer and place your hands properly to give abdominal thrusts, also called the Heimlich maneuver.
3. Give 5 quick abdominal thrusts.
4. Repeat sets of 5 abdominal thrusts until the object is expelled or the golfer becomes unconscious.
5. Direct someone to call 911 or your local emergency number.

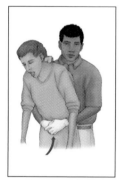

In the Unconscious State

To care for an unconscious golfer who is choking:

1. Check for responsiveness by tapping the golfer's shoulder and loudly asking, "Are you OK?" If the golfer does not respond, direct someone to call 911 or your local emergency number immediately.
2. Tilt the golfer's head back and lift the chin.
3. Check for breathing by looking at the rise and fall of the chest, listening for breath sounds, and feeling for breaths on your cheek.

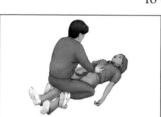

4. If the golfer is not breathing, give 2 slow breaths. If the first breath does not go in, retilt the head and try a second breath.
5. If breaths still do not go in, give up to 5 abdominal thrusts (Heimlich maneuver).
6. Perform a finger sweep in the mouth.
7. Open the airway and give a breath.
8. If breath does not go in, retilt the head and try a second breath. If unsuccessful, repeat cycles of 5 thrusts, finger sweep, and breaths.

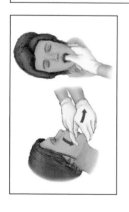

9. If breaths go in, check for a neck pulse.
10. If the neck pulse is present but the golfer is not breathing, give 1 slow breath every 5 seconds for anyone over the age of 8 years. (It would be 1 breath every 3 seconds for a child age 8 years and younger.) Watch and see if the golfer's chest is rising and falling with each breath.
11. If the golfer has no neck pulse, start CPR (see Appendix).

Cold-Related Emergencies

Golfing in cool or cold weather can lead to a lower-than-normal body temperature (hypothermia).

Signs that a golfer is suffering from the cold are red or swollen skin, skin cool to the touch, and lack of shivering in a golfer who has become wet and remained wet for a prolonged period of time.

PROTECT YOURSELF

First aid kits normally contain disposable medical exam gloves and a mouth-to-barrier device. To prevent the spread of infectious airborne and bloodborne diseases, it is recommended that you use these body substance isolation devices.

To care for a golfer who has a cold-related injury:
1. Stop the heat loss! Handling the golfer very gently, remove him or her from the cold environment.
2. Remove and replace wet clothing with dry clothing or blankets.
3. Cover the golfer's head. Fifty percent of body heat is lost through the head.
4. If the golfer is unconscious, check pulse for 30 to 45 seconds to determine if CPR is needed.

Diabetic Emergencies

Occasionally, the prolonged exposure to heat, extended hours of exercise, and performance anxiety that comes with playing golf can trigger an emergency for a diabetic.

Signs to look for in a person who is having a diabetes-related emergency are sudden loss of coordination, staggering, anger, pale skin, confusion, excessive sweating, and trembling.

To care for a golfer who has a known diabetic condition:

1. Check for altered mental status (he or she may appear intoxicated, be staggering, or be unconscious)
2. If the golfer is conscious, offer a food or drink containing sugar. Some examples are table sugar, soda, candy, or fruit juice.
3. If he or she is not better in 10 to 15 minutes, call 911 or your local emergency number.

Eye Injuries

Foreign objects in the eye are the most frequent eye injury and can be very painful.

Signs to look for in a person who has an eye injury are visible object in the eye like sand or dirt, tearing, and redness of the eye.

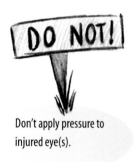

Don't apply pressure to injured eye(s).

To care for a golfer with a loose object in the eye:

1. Pull the lower eyelid down and have the golfer look up.
2. If you see the object, remove it by flushing the eye with water, or patting it gently with a clean, moist cloth or sterile dressing.
3. If the golfer has trouble keeping the eye open, lift the upper eyelid over a matchstick or cotton-tipped swab. If you can see the object, remove it by flushing the eye with water, or patting it gently with a clean, moist cloth or sterile dressing.
4. Sand under a contact lens can abrade the surface of the eye. To prevent serious damage, the lens should be removed and the eye flushed with water or a wetting solution.

To care for a golfer with a fixed object in the eye:
Call 911 or your local emergency number immediately.

1. Do not remove the object.
2. Protect the eye to prevent the object from being driven in deeper. If one eye moves, the second eye also moves, so cover both eyes.

To care for a golfer with a chemical or pesticide in the eye:

1. Call 911 or your local emergency number immediately.
2. Hold the injured eye open.
3. Flush the open eye with water for 15 to 20 minutes.
4. Turn the golfer's head to the side so that the injured eye is below the uninjured eye. In this position, the water will flush the chemical away from the unaffected eye.
5. Loosely bandage the eye.

Fainting

Causes of fainting include hyperventilation, dehydration, low blood sugar, heart attack, epilepsy, heart disease, blood loss, and psychological stress. Some golfers will have early warning signs and/or symptoms of an impending fainting episode. These signs and symptoms include nausea, weakness, chills, abdominal pain, and a pounding headache. With some exceptions, fainting is rarely serious, and in most cases, self-corrects after a few short moments.

Signs to look for in a golfer who has fainted or feels faint are pale skin, sweating, swaying on feet, and falling.

To care for a golfer who feels faint:

1. Have him or her lie down and raise the legs eight to twelve inches. Use a golf bag for this.
2. Monitor breathing and consciousness.
3. Loosen any tight clothing.
4. Apply a cool, wet cloth to forehead and neck.
5. If the golfer is not injured, help him or her sit up.

To care for a golfer who is unconscious but still breathing:

1. Roll him or her onto one side to keep the airway clear.
2. Loosen any tight clothing.
3. Check for injuries.

Call 911 or your local emergency number if
- the golfer has fainted several times.

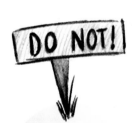

If a golfer faints,
- don't splash or pour water onto an golfer's face to revive him or her.
- don't use smelling salts or ammonia inhalants.
- don't slap the golfer's face.
- don't give the golfer anything to drink unless he or she is conscious, can sit up, and can swallow.

- he or she does not quickly regain consciousness.
- he or she fainted while sitting or lying down.
- he or she faints for no apparent reason.

Head Injuries

Anyone who has been unresponsive because of a head injury, however briefly, must not walk or be left unattended because bleeding inside the skull can occur during the next few hours and result in disorientation or even a coma.

I know I'm getting better at golf, because I'm hitting fewer spectators.

President Gerald Ford

Signs to look for in a golfer with a head injury are blood or watery fluid leaking from an ear or nose and bleeding from the scalp.

To care for a golfer with a head injury:
1. Lay him or her flat and minimize movement of the head and neck.
2. Call 911 or your local emergency number immediately.

If the scalp is bleeding:
1. Control bleeding with direct pressure.
2. For a shallow scalp wound, wash with soap and water

If there is swelling and pain:
1. Apply an ice pack for 15 to 20 minutes.

If the golfer is motionless:
1. Check breathing and pulse.
2. If he or she vomits, roll onto one side to keep the airway open and to drain the fluids out of the mouth.

Heat-Related Emergencies

The higher the humidity, the lower the temperature at which risk of heat-related illnesses begins.

Signs to look for in a person with a heat-related emergency are sweating, flu-like symptoms, hot skin, vomiting, and cramps.

To care for a golfer affected by the heat:
1. Move him or her to a cool place.
2. Have him or her lie down and raise the legs from eight to twelve inches. Use your golf bag or cart.

3. Remove excess clothing.
4. If the golfer is conscious and not nauseated, offer a drink of cool water or a commercial electrolyte drink.
5. Sponge him or her with cool water or fan the body.
6. Call 911 or your local emergency number if the golfer is unconscious, or if the condition does not improve within 30 minutes.

Lightning Strikes

Injuries from lightning can take a number of forms. The most immediate life-threatening dangers are heart failure and brain damage.

Signs to look for in a person who may have been struck and injured by lightning are burns or wounds to the skin, seizures, or unconsciousness.

To care for a golfer who has been struck by lightning:
1. Call 911 or your local emergency number immediately— this could be a life-threatening situation.
2. Check for consciousness, breathing, and a pulse.
3. If pulseless, begin CPR and use an automatic external defibrillator (AED) if available.
4. Keep the golfer warm.

Nosebleeds

Nosebleeds are fairly common and sometimes associated with golfers who take a blood-thinning medication such as aspirin. Begin caring for a golfer's nosebleed by directing him or her in administering self-care to control the bleeding. This will reduce your chances of coming into direct contact with the golfer's blood. Also, help the golfer limit the amount of blood that drains down the throat and into the stomach. This will reduce the chances of vomiting, which could block the airway.

To care for a golfer with a nosebleed:
1. Wear gloves.
2. Have the golfer sit down and lean slightly forward.
3. Have the golfer pinch his or her nostrils together at the bridge of the nose.
4. Have the golfer maintain this pressure for at least 5 minutes. Then have him or her slowly release the pressure, and determine if clotting has been successful. If bleeding continues, have the golfer reapply pressure to the nostrils.

5. If the bleeding cannot be controlled, or if the golfer has complained of any related medical problems, such as head injury, send someone to the pro shop to call 911.

Seizures

Although there are many causes of seizures, emergency treatment includes the same basic steps. Signs to look for in a person having a seizure are a blank stare, a sudden cry followed by a fall, rigid appearance, muscle jerks, and unconsciousness.

To care for a golfer who has had or is having a seizure:
1. Remove nearby objects to prevent injury.
2. Turn the golfer onto his or her side, if possible.
3. After seizure stops, keep the golfer on the side and offer your help. Most seizures are not emergencies.
4. Call 911 or your local emergency number when
   • the seizure lasts for more than five minutes.
   • the golfer does not have a known seizure disorder.
   • the golfer is not wearing a medical-alert identification tag.
   • the golfer is slow to recover.
   • you can see any signs of injury or illness.
   • the golfer is pregnant.

Snake Bites

Only four snake species in the United States are poisonous: rattlesnakes, copperheads, water moccasins (copperheads), and coral snakes. If you are not certain whether a snake is poisonous, assume it is venomous.

Signs to look for in a person bitten by a snake are swelling and fang marks at the site of the bite. A life-threatening systemic reaction and shock may occur.

To care for a golfer who has had snake bite:
1. Call 911 or your local emergency number.
2. Keep the victim still. Walking actively increases venom absorption.
3. If safely possible, identify the snake (i.e., size, color, markings).
4. Clean the snake bite site.
5. Immobilize any injured limb (i.e., sling or splint an arm or hand).
6. If the bite has just occured and you're more than one hour away from medical treatment, use a snake bite kit with a suction device to extract venom.

Spinal Injuries

Any golfer who has sustained injuries from a fall or from a vehicular accident should be checked for a spinal injury before being moved.

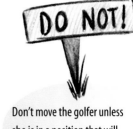

Signs to look for in a golfer with a spinal injury are loss of bodily functions, deformities (odd-looking angle of the golfer's head and neck), no feeling when pinching the fingers or toes, inability to wiggle fingers or toes, and inability to squeeze your hand or push his or her foot against it.

Don't move the golfer unless she is in a position that will endanger her further.

To care for a golfer whom you suspect has a spinal injury:
1. Call or direct someone to call 911 or your local emergency number immediately.
2. Keep the injured person still.
3. Stay with the golfer until EMS personnel arrive with the proper equipment to move him or her.
4. Check for breathing and pulse.

Ticks

Tick bites are nearly painless, so the tick attachment is not usually noticed until later. Signs to look for in a person with an embedded tick are swelling, redness, a blood-filled tick attached to skin, and part of a tick sticking out of the skin.

To care for a golfer with an embedded tick:
1. Gently pull the tick out with tweezers. Grasp the tick's head as close to the skin as possible—a small piece of the golfer's skin may also be removed.
2. Wash the bite site with soap and water.
3. Apply rubbing alcohol to the area to disinfect it.
4. Apply an ice pack to the area to reduce pain.
5. In young golfers, inform the golfer's parents or guardians of the incident. Ask them to watch for signs of infection or symptoms such as severe headache, fever, and rash. These symptoms may develop at any time from 3 to 30 days after the incident. If any of these symptoms occur, the parents should seek medical attention immediately.

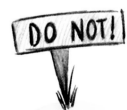

- don't grab the tick at the rear of its body.
- don't twist or jerk the tick while pulling it out.
- don't use any substance to try to remove the tick.

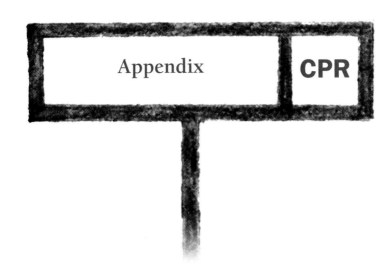

Appendix   CPR

To obtain the skills necessary to resuscitate a person who has stopped breathing, or who is without circulation, you should take a course in cardiopulmonary resuscitation (CPR) given by the National Safety Council (1-800-621-7619) or the American Heart Association. This section provides only the essentials required to start resuscitation until someone with more skill arrives to take over the situation.

Basic Life Support

Basic life support (BLS) refers to lifesaving procedures that focus on the victim's airway, breathing, and circulation. BLS includes rescue breathing, CPR, and obstructed airway management.

Basic life support is most effective when it is started quickly, is given skillfully, and includes electrical defibrillation.

Resuscitation has two parts: rescue breathing (artificial respirations) and chest compressions. When both are used together they constitute cardiopulmonary resuscitation. Not everyone requires CPR; some victims require only rescue breathing.

WHAT TO LOOK FOR

- Open the airway and check for breathing.
- Check pulse (circulation).
- Confirm that the person is not breathing, has no pulse, and is motionless and unresponsive. (If he or she is moving and responsive, check breathing and pulse a second time.)

When to Start CPR

Start CPR on a motionless person whose breathing and pulse have stopped.

WHAT TO DO

- ◼ Logroll the person onto his or her back.
- ◼ Use the head-tilt/chin-lift method to open the airway.
- ◼ Check for breathing.
- ◼ If the person is breathing and spinal injury is not suspected, place the person into the recovery position.
- ◼ If the person is not breathing, give 2 slow breaths.
- ◼ If the first breath is unsuccessful, treat as for foreign body airway obstruction. (See Breathing Problems and Choking.)
- ◼ Check pulse (carotid artery at neck).
- ◼ If the person has a pulse but is not breathing, give rescue breaths (1 breath every 5 seconds).
- ◼ If the person does not have a pulse, give CPR (cycles of 15 chest compressions followed by 2 breaths are given to anyone over age eight).
- ◼ If help is available, assign one bystander to provide rescue breaths, while you or another bystander provides the cardiac compressions at a rate of 5 compressions to 1 breath (5:1). Check the person's pulse every minute. Continue resuscitation until more skilled rescuers can take over or until you are exhausted.

CPR Illustrated

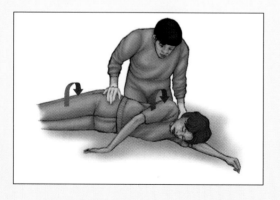

1. Gently roll the person onto his or her back, keeping the head and body in a straight line.

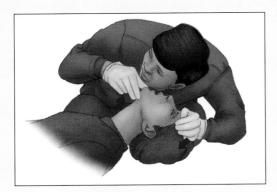

2. Open the airway by tilting the head and lifting the chin (head-tilt/chin-lift technique). Listen and feel for movement of air, and look for rise and fall of chest. If the person is not breathing, give 2 breaths.

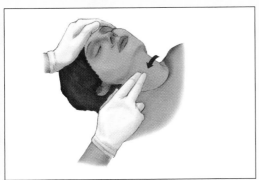

3. Check the carotid pulse in the neck, in the groove next to the Adam's apple. If there is no pulse, begin CPR (chest compressions and rescue breathing).

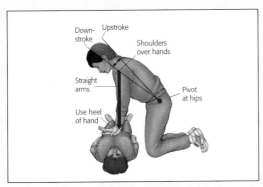

4. Chest compression—15 compressions to 2 breaths

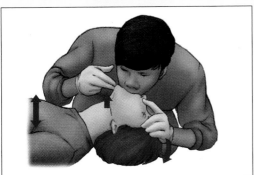

5. Rescue breathing—give 2 breaths

Repeat chest compressions and rescue breathing

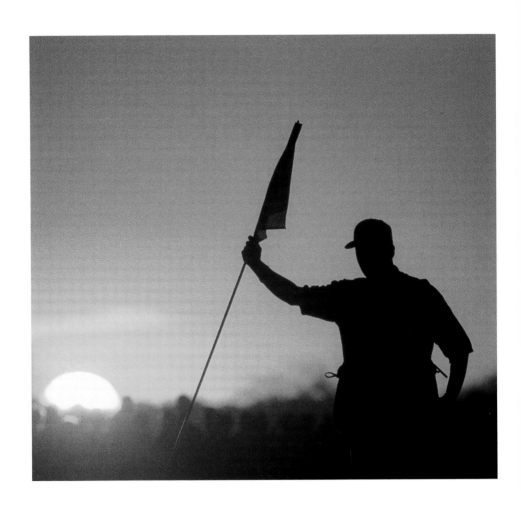

I can sum it up like this—thank God for the game of golf.

—*Arnold Palmer*

Index

A

Acne, leg, 24
Albus, Jim, 107
Alcohol, 38-39
Allergy, 8-12
    decongestant, 10
    immunotherapy, 10-12
    pollen, 8-9
    symptoms, 9, 12, 144
Anaphylactic shock, 144
Angina, 71-72, 75
    symptoms, 77
Animal bite, 144
Antidepressants, 30
Antihistamines, 10
    heat reaction, 30
Anti-inflammatories, 60
Antioxidants, 42
Archer, George, 94
Arthritis, 92-94
Asthma, 131
Attention Deficit Disorder (ADD), 60
Automated external defibrillator (AED), 78-81

B

Back injury, 91, 94-96
Barnes, Brian, 39
Basic life support (BLS), 159
Bee sting, 87, 144
Beta-blocker, 58-59
Birch pollen, 9
Bleeding, 145-146
Blisters, 106-107, 146
Blood pressure, high, 10, 57-58, 122
Boros, Julius, 72, 139
Breathing problem, 148-149
Bunions, 105

C

Caffeine, 37, 39
Calcavecchia, Mark, 97
Calling 911, 143-144
Calories
    consumption, 2
    intake, 34-35

Cancer, skin, 13-15, 17
    melanoma, 20-21
Cardiopulmonary resuscitation (CPR), 78-80, 151, 159-161
Cardiovascular system
    CPR, 78-80, 151
    stress, 3
    walking, 2
Carpal tunnel syndrome, 102
Cart, golf, 4-7
    lightning strike, 52
Centinela Hospital, 109-110
Chausiriporn, Jimmy, 130
Chest pain, 77
Choking, 150-151
Cholesterol level, 1
Claudication, 105
Clearwater, Keith, 97
Clothing, protective, 18-19, 31-32
Club, lightweight, 93
Cold-related emergency, 151
Concentration, 65-66
Confidence, 66-67
Contact lenses, 44-45
Copper bracelet, 41
Corns, 106
Couples, Fred, 91, 109
CPR, 78-80, 151, 159-161
Cramping, 105

D

Daly, John, 38, 109, 130
Daniel, Beth, 97
Decongestant, 10
    heat reaction, 30
Deer tick, 83-85
Delayed onset muscle soreness (DOMS), 104
Dempsey, Garland, 28
Dermatitis, 23
Dey, Joe, 26
Diabetes, 134-137, 151-152
Dichard, Dick, 7
Diuretics, 30, 57-58
Drepanos, Mike, 132

R

Rabies, 144
Ragweed pollen, 8-9
RICE guidelines, 147
Ritalin, 60
Rockwell, Dennis, 54
Rocky Mountain spotted fever, 85
Rodriguez, Chi Chi, 72
Rossburg, Bob, 72-73

S

Salt tablets, 30
See You at the Top, 67
Seizure, 156
Senior golfers
    injuries, 92
    stretching and warm-up, 119
Shoes, 106
Shoulder injury, 97-98
Skin damage, 13-24
    poison ivy, oak, and sumac, 22-23
    protective clothing, 18-19
    skin cancer, 13-15, 17, 20-21
    sunscreen, 14-17
Snake bite, 88, 156
Snead, Sam, 44, 68, 69
Sorenstam, Annika, 46
Spider bite, 87
Spinal injury, 157
Steere, Alan, 82
Steroids, 10, 63
Stewart, Payne, 60, 91, 94
Stockton, Dave, 119
Strange, Curtis, 66, 111
Strength training, 110-113
    junior golfers, 130-131
    women golfers, 121, 124-127
Stress, 3, 68-69
Stretching, 115-119
Sugar intake, 36
Sunglasses, 20, 46-48
Sunscreen, 14-17

T

Tendonitis, 91, 102-103
Tick bite, 83-85, 157
Toledo, Esteban, 67

Tranquilizers, 30
Trevino, Lee, 52, 66, 109-110
Tschetter, Kris, 45
Turner, Sherri, 134

V

Van Houten, Jack, 80
Venturi, Ken, 4, 25-27, 102
Verplank, Scott, 134
Victim Assessment, 143
    See specific injury
Visualization, 67-68
Vitamins, 35-36
    antioxidants, 42

W

Walking, 1-7
    caloric consumption, 2
    and cholesterol levels, 1
    and stress, 3
Warm-up, 115-119
Watson, Tom, 4
Weather, 25-32
    cold-related emergency, 151
    drug reactions, 30
    heart conditions, 76
    heat exhaustion, 28-31, 154-155
    lightning, 51-55, 155
    protective clothing, 31-32
Webb, Kerri, 103
Weight lifting, 111
Women golfers, 121-127
    menopause, 123
    pregnancy, 121-123
    strength training, 121, 124-127
Wrist injury, 102-103

Y

"Yips," 69-70

Z

Ziglar, Zig, 67
Zoeller, Fuzzy, 66

References

1. Palank, E. A., Hargraves, E. H. "Benefits of Walking the Golf Course: Effects on Lipoprotein Levels and Risk Ratios." *Physician and Sports Medicine* 18, 10 (1990): 77.

2. Vallbona, C., Hazelwood, C., Jurida, G., "Response of Pain to Static Magnetic Fields in Postpolio Patients: A Double-Blind Pilot Study." *Archives of Physical Medicine and Rehabilitation* 78, 11 (1997): 1201-1203.

3. Pavlovic, P., Swanson, D., Tirado, D. "Human Response to Physical Stress Improved by Antioxidants." Abstract, *Proceedings Oxygen Society* (November 20, 1998).

4. Becker, L., Eisenberg, M., Fahrenbruch, C., Cobb, L. "Public Locations of Cardiac Arrest." *Circulation* 97 (1998): 2106-2109.

5. LaPorte, R. E., Dorman, J. S., Tajima, N., et al. "Pittsburgh Insulin-Dependent Diabetes Mellitus Morbidity and Mortality Study: Physical Activity and Diabetic Complications." *Pediatrics* 78, 6 (1986): 1027-1033.

6. Smith, S. "Duck! You Dummy..." *Golf Digest* (June 1999): 105-112.

Credits

p. iv   © Ed Chappell
p. 5   © Jim Cummins / FPG International
p. 14   Courtesy of the American Academy of
         Dermatologists (AAD)
p. 18   Cynthia Strohmeyer, MD
p. 21   Courtesy of the American Academy
         of Dermatologists (AAD)
p. 33   Michael O'Leary/Tony Stone Images
p. 37   Ed Palank
p. 51   Courtesy of Xtreme Research Corporation
p. 56   Ed Palank
p. 81   Jose Salazar (all)
p. 95   Linda DeBruyn
p. 96   Linda DeBruyn (all)
p. 97   Linda DeBruyn (all)
p. 98   Linda DeBruyn (t)
p. 98   Linda DeBruyn (m)
p. 100   Linda DeBruyn (all)
p. 101   Linda DeBruyn (all)
p. 102   Paul Chesley/© Tony Stone Images
p. 108   Linda DeBruyn (t)
p. 112   Larry Newell (m)
p. 112   Larry Newell (b)
p. 132   Joan Drepanos

The following material was provided by the
New York Times Company Magazine Group, Inc.
Copyright ©1999 New York Times Company
Magazine Group, Inc. All rights reserved.

p. viii   Rusty Jarrett
p. xi   Stephen Szurlej
p. xvi   David W. Harbaugh
p. 3   David W. Harbaugh
p. 9   Jim Moriarty
p. 11   Marcus Hamilton
p. 17   Jim Moriarty
p. 19   Dom Furore
p. 20   Bob Ewell
p. 26   Ken Regan
p. 27   Jim Moriarty
p. 29   Larry Lambrecht
p. 38   Rusty Jarrett
p. 41   Stephen Szurlej
p. 45   Bob Ewell (l)
p. 45   Stephen Szurlej (r)
p. 47   Stephen Szurlej
p. 47   Golf Digest (b)
p. 50   Bob Ewell

p. 53   Stephen Szurlej
p. 59   Golf Digest
p. 61   Stephen Szurlej
p. 64   Golf Digest
p. 67   Gary Newkirk
p. 72   Stephen Szurlej
p. 87   Marc Rosenthal
p. 89   Rusty Jarrett
p. 90   David W. Harbaugh
p. 91   Stephen Szurlej
p. 91   Eddie Dibbs (x-ray)
p. 94   Golf Digest
p. 98   David W. Harbaugh (b)
p. 104   Dee Darden
p. 106   Stephen Szurlej
p. 110   Scott Halleran
p. 113   Bob Ewell
p. 116   Jim Moriarty (all)
p. 117   Jim Moriarty (all)
p. 118   Jim Moriarty (all)
p. 119   Jim Moriarty
p. 120   Stephen Szurlej
p. 122   Dean Batchelder
p. 124   Dom Furore (all)
p. 125   Dom Furore (all)
p. 126   Dom Furore (all)
p. 127   Dom Furore
p. 128   E.H. Wallop
p. 135   Stephen Szurlej
p. 137   Stephen Szurlej
p. 138   Larry Lambrecht
p. 163   Gary Newkirk

Photo captions on pages 116-119 were adapted
from material provided by the New York Times
Company Magazine Group, Inc. Photo captions
on pages 124-127 are from material provided by
the New York Times Company Magazine Group,
Inc. Copyright ©1999 New York Times Company
Magazine Group, Inc. All rights reserved.